Counselling

A Guide to Practice in Nursing

For Sally, Aaron and Rebecca

Other books by the same author

Learning Human Skills: An Experiential Guide for Nurses:
2nd Edition

Professional and Ethical Issues for Nurses
(with C. M. Chapman)

Counselling Skills for Health Professionals

Teaching Interpersonal Skills: An Experiential Handbook for Health Professionals

Nurse Education: The Way Forward
(with C. M. Chapman)

Nursing Research in Action: Developing Basic Skills
(with P. Morrison)

Experiential Learning in Action

Coping With Stress in the Health Professions

Know Yourself: A Handbook of Self-Awareness Activities for Nurses

Effective Communication Skills for Health Professionals

Communicate!: A Guide to Communication Skills for Health Workers

Caring and Communicating: The Interpersonal Relationship in Nursing
(with P. Morrison)

Caring and Communicating: The Interpersonal Relationship in Nursing: Facilitators' Manual
(with P. Morrison)

Aspects of AIDS Counselling

Counselling

A Guide to Practice in Nursing

Philip Burnard
PhD, MSc, RGN, RMN, DipN, Cert Ed, RNT,

Director of Postgraduate Nursing Studies, University of Wales College of Nursing, Cardiff, Wales, UK; and Honorary Lecturer in Nursing Studies, Hogeschool Midden Nederland, Utrecht, The Netherlands

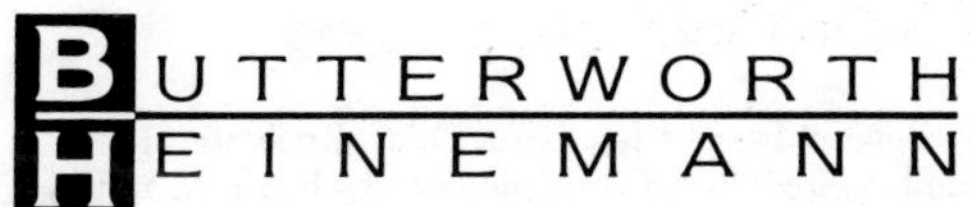

Butterworth-Heinemann Ltd
Linacre House, Jordan Hill, Oxford OX2 8DP

 PART OF REED INTERNATIONAL BOOKS

OXFORD LONDON BOSTON
MUNICH NEW DELHI SINGAPORE SYDNEY
TOKYO TORONTO WELLINGTON

First published 1992

British Library Cataloguing in Publication Data
Burnard, Philip
Counselling: A Guide to Practice in Nursing
I. Title
610.73

ISBN 0 7506 0643 6

Composition by Genesis Typesetting, Laser Quay, Rochester, Kent
Printed and bound in Great Britain by Biddles Ltd, Guildford and King's Lynn

Contents

Introduction

This book is for any nurse who works with patients. Patients, like all of us, have a variety of problems. Nurses often feel that they cannot talk to those patients. The aim of this book is to help you to become a more effective listener. It is also aimed at making you more effective when you talk to patients. It is hoped that it will also help you in your conversations with friends and colleagues.

Part of the problem of coping with people's anxieties is that we do not always know what to say. This book will not tell you what to say but it will help you to develop the skills to decide.

What this book will not do is turn you into a psychotherapist. It does not offer an explicit psychological perspective, although it acknowledges that we all work from one. It will, however, help you to clarify your own beliefs about people and about problems.

This book contains a straightforward model of counselling – although counselling, itself, is rarely straightforward. Why a 'model' of counselling in nursing? Models are everywhere. Most nurses have read or used models of nursing. Model, here, is used to denote a plan of action, a map or a way of working with patients in a systematic way, through counselling. I have found that the development of *structure* makes most things a bit easier. That is all that this model offers: structure in the therapeutic process. It also offers a range of skills to go with that structure. In essence, this model is a *descriptive* one: it seeks to clarify what the counselling relationship may be and how it may be structured.

Also within this book is a 'model within a model'. I have developed a way of counselling at three levels: the feeling level, the thinking level and the concrete level. This is also discussed in the book as a practical aid to exploring problems.

The range of skills described in this book have developed from a number of sources. First, they have developed out of my own training as a counsellor, researcher and educator over the past 20 years. Second, they have been developed out of the theory and practice of counselling as it is described in other textbooks and through the research into the topic. Certain writers have been particularly influential in my thinking and a short list would include: Jean-Paul Sartre, Carl Rogers, B. F. Skinner, Eric Fromm, George Kelly, Victor Frankl and John Heron. References to these and other writers can be found in the bibliography at the end of this book.

Finally, the skills have developed out of my own research and thinking on the topic. I do not believe that there is *one* way to do things. Nor do I believe that any one psychological theory exactly fits the human condition. Psychologists stand guilty of oversimplifying the human situation. We are all very complicated.

None of us likes to think that we are exactly like the next person. I doubt that we are like the next person. Therefore, the ideas in this book and the structure that is offered is *not* the last word on counselling in nursing. It does offer one approach to the process of helping other people. It does this by avoiding a large amount of psychology which, I find, often gets in the way. I prefer to follow the principle outlined by George Kelly (1955): 'If you want to know what someone is about, ask them, they might just tell you.'

This, for me, is an important principle. Rather than developing a range of possible theories about *why* a person is the way that he or she is, it is more important that we hear *that person's* story. In the end, no amount of theorizing on our part is going to change the fact that here we are, faced by another person who is in distress and who, for the moment, is not able to cope with that distress. What is important, it seems to me, is to be able to help that other person to talk through his or her situation, explore it, examine it and, finally, to decide on a course of action.

Thus this book starts from the position that we all do things differently and we all think and feel differently. That is not to say that we are all totally unique. There are lots of ways in which we are similar to each other, too. If that were not true we could neither communicate with each other nor could we develop any theories about the person. I have tried, though, to keep psychological theory to the minimum in this book. I have aimed, instead, at offering a practical and usable model of developing a counselling relationship in nursing. I hope you will not read it as *the* book on counselling, but I do hope that it will help you to think about your relationships with your patients, your friends and colleagues, and with yourself. For we carry ourselves with us wherever we go. We offer ourselves to our patients. We cannot, in the end, hide behind the role of nurse. We have to put up with ourselves even when we do not like ourselves very much.

In summary, this book is a practical account of some strategies for helping you to help your patients, your colleagues and your friends. Those strategies take practice and need to be grounded in your own experience. To that end, you will find exercises and activities here. You will also find an extensive bibliography of references to other books and journals. Further reading, further thinking and further research are essential. This book, like all others, is a moment in time. It is neither the last word nor the definitive model. I believe, though, that the model offered here, works.

I have tried, above all things, to keep it simple and to keep it practical. As I have suggested above, I have not tried to develop an overarching theory of the person nor have I sought to offer a therapy course. There are plenty of other books which do that and some of them are to be found in the bibliography. Above all things, nursing is a practical activity. Listening and talking are also practical activities. Our theories about human beings may be interesting, but our patients usually need something more direct, personal and practical. Counselling, like all other nursing activities, is a practical one.

I have tried to keep the references to a minimum; not because I do not appreciate other people's writing and research – I am dependent upon it. I do feel, however, that a page littered with references is more difficult to read that one which is not. Where I have used other people's work directly, then I have inserted a reference. I have not used references just to decorate the text. I believe that readers can easily work through the bibliography to find the further reading that they need.

There are plenty of well-referenced books already on the shelves. This one is an attempt to put into words practical helping processes. It is also an attempt to simplify and clarify what is at once a simple and difficult task. That task is that of helping another human being to face, come to terms with and solve some of their personal problems. A huge task, put like that! The structure, though, can make the task easier: thus, this book.

What is in this book?

The book offers a straightforward account of the counselling process in nursing. It is not an elaborate account. It does, however, cover all the stages that can be worked through to enable a nurse to work in a therapeutic way with patients, colleagues and friends. It is my contention that we are *all* counsellors. We all help others with their problems. That is not to say that we are all psychotherapists or psychoanalysts but simply that we are often of great help and comfort to others through the simple process of listening and of not getting in the way. This book describes ways in which these simple processes can be enhanced.

The book is clearly structured. After early chapters offering definitions, some theory and basic information about counselling, there are chapters on each of thc stages of the model. Each stage also offers specific skills which are described. Also, each stage is illustrated by specific examples, drawn from nursing/counselling practice and is accompanied by activities for developing the skills described. How these activities can be used is discussed below. The book closes with a chapter about teaching counselling skills, a list of useful addresses, a counselling skills self-assessment rating scale and a detailed bibliography of further reading.

I believe that we learn best from direct, personal experience. I also believe that we have to put ideas into practice and we have to see that they work. The emphasis, in this book, is always on the practical application of each stage of the model.

The word 'nurse' has been used to denote the person doing the counselling. This can be read as health visitor, manager or educator as required. I hope that the book will also be of use to other health professionals including midwives. I have used the word 'client' as the label for the person on the receiving end of counselling. It is not an ideal term but I hope that it covers patients, residents, customers as well as friends and colleagues.

Whom is the book for?

As I suggested at the outset, this book is for almost all nurses. More particularly, it will be of use to the following groups of people:

- Nursing students
- Graduate and postgraduate student nurses
- Clinical nurses both trained and untrained
- Community nurses
- Nurses who work in specialist units such as ICU and AIDS units
- Nurse educators
- Nurse managers
- Voluntary workers
- Anyone else who is interested in becoming more effective in their helping relationships with others.

How do I use the book?

Like any other, the book can be read through at one or more sittings. It can also be worked through as part of a group activity. This latter approach is particularly valuable if the aim is to learn how to counsel. Most chapters contain simple experimential learning activities which are designed to reinforce the issues discussed. They are best carried out in a supportive group.

The last chapter of the book is explicitly for those who have a training role. It will be of interest, though, to others who are in training or who are studying counselling training or interpersonal skills training for it offers a rationale and a method for using the activities at the end of each chapter.

The experiential approach to developing counselling skills

We all learn from experience. Also, we do not *always* learn from experience. We probably only learn when we reflect on what happens to us. We have to notice what happens in order to learn. Otherwise, the experience just happens to us and we are none the wiser. We have to be present when things happen and we have to notice their happening. This process is known as experiential learning.

The concept of experiential learning is discussed in the final chapter of this book, but it is important to say a few things about it here. First, from the research that I have done, I have found that for some people, the terms 'experiential learning' and 'role play' are not popular ones. Not everyone likes to learn through elaborate group activities. On the other hand, no one learns anything about counselling simply by reading about it. There has to be a happy medium. A mixture of theoretical input and skills rehearsal seems to strike that balance. Also, we can learn a lot simply by observing ourselves at work. This, too, is experiential learning.

I often refer to this sort of experiential learning in this book for I believe that we all can and do learn much about ourselves and others by simply noticing ourselves in this way. Role play and group activities help some people but not all. The 'learning' from role play is not always transferred over into the real world of nursing. Noticing, as I have described it here, is part of learning through living and can do much to make us more aware of our strengths and deficits in the interpersonal domain.

1

Counselling in nursing

What is counselling?

Counselling is something that all nurses do. It is probably something that everyone does. Right from the start, it is important to demystify the process for if we do not, there is a danger that we might miss some important chances to help others.

Counselling has been defined in many ways in many books. Most definitions offer variations around the following key points. Counselling involves:

- Two people, one of whom is identified as a counsellor and the other who can be called the client
- The helping of the client by the counsellor
- A situation in which the client has problems, sometimes clearly identified and sometimes not, which he or she shares with the counsellor
- A relationship that is different to plain conversation and yet is not psychotherapy.

The main aim of the chapter is to explore some of these issues and to try to identify what counselling in nursing might be. As was stressed in the Introduction, this is not the last word on counselling, but one approach to it. It is important to read widely on the topic and to compare different approaches. The approach offered in this book presupposes that all nurses are capable of helping other people with their problems and that counselling is essentially a *practical* enterprise in that its aim is problem solving.

What is a therapeutic relationship?

We all have a variety of relationships with a variety of different people. We may have formal, work-related relationships with colleagues, for example. We have closer relationships of a different sort, with parents and members of the family. We have relationships that are closer still, and yet different again, with friends and those with whom we fall in love.

I am using the term 'therapeutic relationship' to describe the sort of relationship that occurs in counselling. There is no doubt that the relationship is central to counselling. Patterson (1985) says this on the subject: 'Counselling or psychotherapy is an interpersonal relationship. Note that I don't say that counselling or psychotherapy involves an interpersonal relationship – it *is* an interpersonal relationship.'

The therapeutic relationship is almost paradoxical for it is close and yet professional. It is warm and genuine and yet you do not fall in love with the other person. You care for them and yet not in the way that you do about your family. Most of all, the therapeutic relationship is a *helping* relationship in which the counsellor is helping the client.

Of course, it is not always as simple as this. We are often helped by our clients. We often learn as much about ourselves when counselling as we do about the other person. But the point is that the counsellor's *intention* in counselling is to be helpful and thus therapeutic for the other person. You do not set out in counselling to sort out your own problems. You do not set out in counselling to sort out other person's problems either, but you do start with the aim of helping the other person in her struggle. This, then, is the therapeutic relationship. It can be characterized in the following ways:

- There is an intention on the part of the counsellor to help
- The relationship is of benefit to the client
- The counsellor cares about the client
- The relationship is reciprocated to some degree but, in the end, it is the client's needs which are uppermost
- The relationship is always an ethical one and is not exploited by the counsellor.

The last two issues are vital. Not all therapeutic relationships are necessarily reciprocal ones. That is to say, it is not always the case that the counsellor and client *both* feel close to one another. Certainly, the pair do not share all of their problems in a reciprocal way.

Also, the relationship is bound to be an ethical one. The client must be able to trust the counsellor and the counsellor must always act as a professional person. After all, the client is sharing important and personal information with the counsellor and a close relationship often results from this sharing. It is essential, if the relationship is to remain therapeutic (and not become some other sort of relationship) that the counsellor always acts in the best interests of the client and according to that person's wishes.

Counselling or psychotherapy?

This book is not about psychotherapy. Psychotherapy is an umbrella term for a wide range of therapies that are usually used to help people who are suffering from mental ill health, who want to solve some fairly deep-seated personal problems, or who feel that they want to develop themselves through a therapeutic relationship. Examples of the varieties of psychotherapy include:

- Psychoanalysis
- Behaviour therapy
- Gestalt therapy
- Transactional analysis
- Group therapy
- Reichian body work
- Hypnotherapy, etc.

Normally, a psychotherapist has had a fairly lengthy and intense training. Most psychotherapists have also been in therapy themselves as this is considered necessary for the development of the personal and technical skills required to be a therapist.

Another way of looking at the differences between psychotherapy and counselling is to consider that psychotherapy is a much 'heavier' sort of process than is counselling. That is to say that the psychotherapist encourages the client to dig deeper into his or her feelings than is usually the case in counselling and to explore the client's world in much more detail.

While the sort of counselling advocated in this book also takes into account the client's feelings, the idea of *in depth* exploration of this sort is not discussed. Any nurse who wants to take up psychotherapy should consider formal training. Oddly, though, no one *has* to train as a psychotherapist in order to call themselves one. This has led to a few people undertaking very short trainings and then practising as psychotherapists. It would be hard to justify this sort of approach, given the fragility of other human beings. Anyone seeking psychotherapy would be well advised to check the credentials and training of the person offering therapy.

When is it counselling and when is it friendship?

Why have counselling at all? Surely most of us can talk things over with our friends? By and large, for most of us who are not in hospital or not suffering in some way, this is true. If I have problems with my life, I tend to discuss them with my wife or my friends. Sometimes, though, this is not enough. Sometimes, there are no friends to talk things over with. Sometimes, friends are not sure what to say, become judgemental or get fed up with you. It is at this point that the counsellor can help.

Also, the counsellor purposely sets out, as we have seen, to offer a *therapeutic relationship*. It would be stretching a point to suggest that all friendships are based around this idea. Mostly, friendships involve an exchange of thoughts, feelings, ideas and problems on a fairly mutual basis. The point about the therapeutic conversation and about counselling is that the relationship is always geared in one direction – towards the client. The client is always the focal and central point of the relationship.

The question arises as to whether or not it is possible to be both friend and counsellor. Reflection on our own relationships will suggest that it probably is possible. If I think of my friends, I can see that for much of the time, we are just friends. Every so often though, one of us has a range of problems which needs to be talked through. Sometimes, when this happens, the friend temporarily adopts the role of counsellor. After the problems have been discussed, the relationship evens out again and we revert simply to friends.

So it is in nursing. Sometimes, we are just nurses to our patients or clients. At other times, we switch into the role of counsellor in order to help the other person with problems or feelings. This changing nature of the nursing relationship is not particularly new. Some nurses have always been good at helping people with personal problems. What is new is that more and more people in the profession are appreciating that the counselling role is an essential part of the total role of the nurse. If we really want to offer holistic care, then we need to be able to address the patients' problems and emotions as well as their illnesses and treatments. So, too, if we want to be supportive to our colleagues and friends, it seems, reasonable to expect that counselling skills will help in that direction too.

Should all nurses counsel?

In a word – yes. As we noted above, the role of the nurse is changing. Project 2000 courses have reflected the changing role of the nurse. Primary nursing, nursing theory and the social sciences literature all stress the need for nurses to care for the whole person – emotional stresses and all. If we are to function as people who care for the whole person, we need to develop those skills specific to do the job.

Some will say that they do not need training: they are 'naturally' good at talking to people. No doubt this is true of some people. The point is that counselling is less about talking to people and much more about *listening*. Throughout this book and at the risk of becoming boring, the emphasis will be on developing listening skills. It is only when we can walk beside the other person, enter their world-view and understand things the way that *they* understand things that we will begin to become effective as counsellors. Listening, then, is the key skill in counselling. We all learned to listen in the first place. We can all learn to do it better.

All this is not to suggest that counselling is *all* that nurses will do. It is not being advocated that nurses be forced to set themselves up as general counsellors and offer help on all sorts of psychological matters. It is merely to note that the sorts of skills that are described in this book and that can safely be called 'counselling skills' are useful to all nurses in all aspects of their work. Counselling skills can enhance communication and caring between nurses and patients, nurses and nurses, and nurses and other colleagues.

In the end, too, they can help us to sort out some of our own problems. For in the end, we are also fragile and in need of help. As obvious as this seems now, it is not so long ago that nurses were expected to be devoid of emotions and devoid of problems. The 'stiff upper lip' was the norm and if you had feelings you were expected to hide them. The atmosphere in nursing is changing. Slowly it is being recognized that we are all human and that we all suffer to some degree. Counselling skills can help to make us more human, more caring and more *able* to care. For it is one thing to *intend* to care and quite another to have the practical skills to be *able* to care.

Nurses and counselling

There is not a long tradition of nurses as counsellors. Nor do nurses necessarily see themselves as fitting into the role of the counsellor. In a recent study of nurses' attitudes towards counselling skills, we found that most nurses tended towards advice giving and prescription rather than towards listening and encouraging (Burnard and Morrison, 1989). In another study, we found that nurses thought themselves far more able to give information and advice than to handle feelings and confrontation (Morrison and Burnard, 1991).

The approach taken in this book is directly contrary to these finding. It is suggested that counselling is much more about listening, encouraging and caring than it is about giving advice and information. Sometimes, of course, it will be necessary to give advice and information. This is rarely the case when it comes to personal problems and feelings. In the domain of *my* problems and feelings, I am the expert. It would be odd to argue otherwise. Could anyone really claim to know what is best for me? Would you like it if someone claimed to know what was best for you? I doubt it. And yet, up and down the country, it is still possible to hear people say things like: 'If I were you, I would . . .' or 'Well, you know what you have to do now. You have to . . .'. The implication is that it *is* possible to be an expert for someone else. This implication is the one that is challenged most strongly in this book. If we want our clients to develop autonomy and personal strength, then we must trust them to be the authority on their own lives.

Basic principles of counselling

From the discussion above, it is possible to draw out some basic principles of counselling in nursing. The list below is not an exhaustive one. It does not cover every possible principle of counselling. It is offered more as a basis for introducing the topic and for discussion. At this stage, the principles are merely offered as they stand. They will be discussed further in later chapters. Read through them and note the degree to which you do or do not accept them.

- The client knows best. He or she is the expert on his or her problems and feelings. In the end, only he or she can make decisions about them
- Interpretation by another person rarely helps. That is to say, it rarely helps to say things like, 'What you *really* mean is . . .' or 'I know you *think* that's true but what is *really* happening is . . .'.
- It is important to enter the client's 'frame of reference'. We all look at the world in a unique sort of way. If we are to begin to understand the other person and to help them, it is vital that we try to view the world as they do.
- Judgement and moralizing are rarely appropriate. What has happened has happened. It is rarely helpful to blame the client or to say, 'I'm not surprised at what has happened . . . why ever did you do that in the first place?'
- Your experience is not the same as the client's. This really is a fundamental rule. It is very easy to for me to begin to compare my life with yours or my experience with your experience, and yet we both have different histories and look at things from different points of view. Therefore, be very careful before you say things like, 'I know just what you mean . . . I'm just like that myself'. One thing is for sure – you are not.
- Listening is the first and last principle of good counselling.

Varieties of counselling in nursing

The question remains – how can nurses use counselling in nursing? There are at least four groups of people that the nurse may find him or herself helping in this way:

- Clients
- Relatives
- Colleagues
- Friends.

Client counselling

There are numerous examples of the ways in which counselling can help clients: as inpatients, outpatients, or as patients in the community. Examples include the following:

- On admission to hospital
- To reduce anxiety prior to surgery
- When the person is worried about life at home
- When the person is feeling particularly stressed.

There are also many occasions on which relatives of patients will be helped by counselling. Examples, here, include:

- Explaining the nature of an operation
- Breaking bad news
- Helping to accept the client's illness.

Colleague counselling

Just as clients in the clinical setting can be helped by counselling, so, too, can colleagues. Such colleagues may include fellow nurses, senior nurses, students, tutors and so forth. What is interesting and challenging is that it is usually easier to counsel 'down' the hierarchy. That is to say that it is easier for a senior nurse to counsel a student than it is for a student to counsel a student. Reasons for this are probably numerous, but the most important one is probably the power relationship between the two parties. It is a reflection on the lack of equality between client and counsellor that this hierarchical issue exists at all.

It is sometimes possible to believe from a reading of the literature on counselling that clients and counsellors share an equal relationship. In practice, this seems rarely to be true. The fact that a person has come to you with problems and has identified you as a counsellor suggests that inequality exists from the first meeting. What is important is that this lack of equality is not exploited nor developed further. Why, then, mention it at all? Merely to note that it exists and that attempts at denying it are probably naive. Once accepted, the difference in status between the two parties need no longer be a problem. Problems *do* exist, however, when there is a pretence of equality.

Educational counselling

Another sort of collegial counselling is that which takes place between tutors or lecturers and their students. At least two subdivisions of types of counselling can be made here. First, there is the straightforward educational counselling of the sort in which discussion takes place about academic progress, essays, clinical placements and any number of other educational issues. They are 'straightforward' in that they represent problems that can usually be worked through by both tutor and student via discussion and negotiation.

In the educational context, the term 'counselling' is sometimes misused or at least used to mean something different to the sense in which it is being used here. It is sometimes used as a euphemism for a disciplinary action or a telling off. A few months ago I was reassured by a clinical ward sister in this way: 'Don't worry about Student Nurse Jones, Dr Burnard, I've given her a bloody good counselling!' The sister was clearly using the word in a different sort of way to the way in which it is being discussed here.

The other sort of educational counselling occurs when the tutor or lecturer acts as a student's personal counsellor. This role may or may not be part of a mentoring programme. Mentoring, supervising or the management of preceptorship is a developing system of support following the introduction of Project 2000 type courses. Sometimes, the tutor or lecturer is called upon to act as the person to whom the student can take personal and life problems.

It is worth the tutor or lecturer considering in some detail whether or not he or she is ideally placed to take on such a role. While many tutors and lecturers may be happy to function in this way and while it may be a replacement for their 'clinical' role, there are difficulties in adopting such a dual role. First, the tutor or lecturer who works both as teacher and as counsellor has to be able to switch comfortably between those roles, as does the student. Sometimes, it is possible to see that there may be a conflict of interests. The teacher who lectures to a class in which the student is present may become hypersensitive to the problems of that student and find him or herself unable to discuss certain issues in the classroom because they so clearly impinge on the problems of the student in question.

Second, there may be a conflict of interests when it comes to marking examination papers of the student concerned. That we become 'involved' with the people we counsel is clear. Whether or not we can then detach ourselves sufficiently to mark papers and course work becomes a fraught question. There are no easy answers here. I have resolved the issue in my own practice by only counselling students who I am not going to examine later in the course. I accept that there are times when I am painfully aware that the topic of conversation in the classroom has painful implications for a particular student, but accept that this is part and parcel of everyday life and that I cannot allow myself to become over protective at the expense of other students. No doubt you will resolve the issue, if it applies to you, in the way that you see fit.

On a visit to various colleges and universities in Canada and the USA a few years ago, I noticed that lecturers there tended to take a much more straightforward line on this issue. Most of the counsellor/lecturers that I met simply refused to see students for personal counselling. In this way, they avoided any of the problems that may occur in this sensitive arena.

Counselling friends

The final example of the way in which nurses can use counselling skills is in the counselling of friends. Clearly, few friends present themselves to us, formally, for counselling. Instead, we find them wanting to talk to us in the pub or asking if we have half an hour in which to talk things over. As we noted above, it is quite possible to switch from the comings and goings of a conversation in a relationship with a friend into a more structured counselling relationship. The skills that are used with clients and colleagues are directly transferable to such situations.

It should be noted, though, that a counselling relationship with a friend is likely to be different to a more 'formal' counselling relationship. This was discussed above a little, under the heading of the 'therapeutic relationship'. The fact is that a relationship between two friends is necessarily different to one between a patient and a nurse. For one thing, two friends already know quite a lot about each other: therefore, the relationship is more 'equal' than it is in a patient/nurse relationship. It may be this factor that sometimes makes counselling friends difficult. Friends often know you so well that they can anticipate the sorts of things you will say, the sorts of beliefs and values that you have, your personal feelings and so on. In the end, if a friend really does want 'objective' counselling, it may be better for them to look elsewhere.

Other sorts of counselling in nursing

There are areas in which specialized counselling is called for. Such counselling often involves information giving and specialized knowledge. Nurses who undertake such counselling usually have special training and examples of counselling of this sort include:

- AIDS counselling
- Genetic counselling
- Counselling people with specific sexual problems
- Counselling people with certain sorts of mental health problems
- Counselling people who are considering abortion
- Counselling people who abuse drugs or alcohol.

Whilst generalizations are always difficult, it is probably best to seek advice about whether or not to engage in counselling people who fall into one or more of the above categories. It is quite possible that you *do* have the expertise to do such counselling, but it is sometimes difficult for us to appreciate what we *do not* know.

What counselling can do

Finally, in this chapter, it is important to identify some of the strengths and limitations of counselling. Counselling is not a panacea: it cannot sort everything out for people. A shortlist of what counselling *can* do, however, would include at least the following:

- Clarifying problem issues
- Relieving tension
- Facilitating problem solving
- Encouraging friendship and companionship
- Ensuring greater clarity of understanding
- Encouraging insight
- Relieving stress.

What counselling cannot do

Counselling has very definite limitations. It is sometimes criticized for the fact that it focuses on the individual and tries to solve problems on an individual basis. People who raise this objection argue that problems do not simply occur within an individual context – they are related to families, partners or to society itself. An example of this would be the person who is depressed because she lives with a partner that she dislikes, in an area of the country that is deprived and is unable to feed and clothe her children because she is unable to work. It would be difficult, in this case, to argue that counselling could solve this person's problems. All counselling might do would be to help her to adjust to her difficulties. Critics might argue that adjustment is likely to stop her from reacting to the personal and social situation that she confronts every day. In this sense, it could be argued that counselling is a 'conservative' process and one that does not address larger social issues.

Other things that counselling cannot do, include:

- Curing mental health problems
- Stopping all suffering
- Turning nurses into psychotherapists
- Solving all problems
- Changing social and political problems.

On the other hand, it might be argued that counselling can help to empower a person to face the political and social difficulties that he or she confronts. Sometimes, personal frustration, anger and pain can get in the way of taking action. Sometimes counselling can help to release some of the feelings that prevent action and open up the way to dealing more directly with some of the larger social issues.

We must know our limitations and stay humble. While counselling can help a wide range of people, there are people it cannot help. It tends to be more effective as an aid to people who can clearly articulate their problems and who are prepared to self-disclose. It is not so easy to counsel those who cannot express themselves. Also, there are times when personality clashes occur and we are unable to help the other person either because they do not like us or us them. In such cases it is important to recognize the impossibility of the situation and find another person to help.

In summary of some of the issues discussed in this chapter, it is possible to identify some of the things that *can* be done in counselling and some that are best avoided.

What not to do in counselling

1 Do not 'interpret' what the patient says.
2 Do not use 'psychobabble'. Keep the language you use plain and simple. For whatever reason, some counsellors adopt a peculiar jargon (e.g. 'May I share something with you?'). Exactly why this happens is not clear. As a general rule, it is better to stick to 'normal' language.
3 Do not attempt psychotherapy.
4 Do not moralize.
5 Do not patronize.
6 Do not argue.
7 Do not automatically compare your experience with the client's.
8 Do not avoid 'referring on' when this is appropriate.

This whole book is about things that you can do in counselling. To start with, though, the following list can be identified.

A shortlist of what to do in counselling

1 Do listen.
2 Do believe what the patient says.
3 Do encourage further talking.
4 Do allow expression of feelings.
5 Do encourage personal problem solving.
6 Do take advice from others when appropriate.
7 Do take care of yourself.

Counselling is a wide-ranging therapeutic approach to helping others. Used wisely and moderately, it can help ease some of the problems of living. All nurses can become better nurses through learning some of the basic skills of counselling. While not all nurses will necessarily seek out people to counsel, all will have occasions on which such skills will be used.

Activities for developing the skills described in this chapter

Activity one: read through the following counselling conversation and note the degree to which it follows the principles discussed in this chapter. Notice what happens when the principles are adhered to and what difference it makes when they are not.

'How are you feeling at the moment?'
'I'm worried, I suppose . . .'
'What are you worried about?'
'My operation. I keep wondering if everything will be OK.'
'I can understand that. I was nervous when I had an operation. It's silly worrying, though, because everything works out alright. I've seen lots of people have the operation your having and I've never known any problems.'
'No, I know it's daft but I'm still anxious about it.'
'What are you particularly worried about?'
'The anaesthetic. You hear some grisly stories about people not coming round. I'm worried about pain afterwards, too. I'm a bit of a coward, I suppose. I guess it will be alright in the end.'
'Have you had an anaesthetic before?'
'Yes. I had my appendix out when I was 12.'
'Did that go OK?'
'Yes. Everything was fine. I had a bit of pain afterwards but nothing I couldn't manage.'
'I had my tonsils out when I was 11. My throat was really sore for about a week. But, like you say, everything goes alright with these operations. But, my throat! I thought I wasn't going to be able to stand it!
'But my operation won't be like that, will it?'
'No. Sorry, I didn't mean to bother you. No, your operation is a straightforward one. Do you know much about it?'
'I know it's not a very long operation and that lots of people have it.'
'Has the doctor talked to you about it?'
'My primary nurse has and she's explained that I will feel a bit uncomfortable for a little while. I don't really know what I'm worrying about really.'
'Do you usually worry about things?'
'I know what is: I don't like leaving the family . . .'
'Leaving the family at home is difficult?'
'Yes. I worry that they won't cope – although I know that they will. I'll be seeing them tonight and I'll talk to them about things. That will make it a bit easier I think. Just talking to you helps. Thanks a lot.'
'Good. Let me know when you want to talk. I'll be free later this evening, about 7.00. If you want to talk then, it'll be fine by me.

The point about most counselling conversations is that they rarely work as they do in books: some of the principles are bound to be ignored. On the other hand, what is noticeable about the above conversation is that when some of the principles *are* put into action, they do encourage the other person to work through his or her feelings. How would you have dealt with this particular conversation? What are the things that you would have done differently? If you can, discuss your thoughts with a colleague.

Activity two: Quilliam and Grove-Stephensen (1991) offer another useful list of things that they consider counselling to be. Read through the list and, from your own experience and from what you have read so far, consider each statement. If you can, discuss the list with a colleague or in a group.

- Counselling is contractual.
- Counselling is caring.
- Counselling is challenging.
- Counselling is explorative.
- Counselling goes from the conscious to the unconscious.
- Counselling is confidential.
- Counselling is conclusive.
- Counselling is empowering.

Questions for reflection and discussion

- To what degree do you think that all nurses should be taught counselling skills?
- Is the distinction between counselling and psychotherapy an unrealistic one or an important one?
- Do Project 2000 courses encourage the development of counselling and interpersonal skills in student nurses?

2

Examples of counselling in nursing

It is important to be clear about what counselling in nursing might be like. In this chapter, some examples of the use of counselling are offered in the form of some case studies that utilize both the principles and some of the skills of counselling.

Case studies of counselling in nursing

The purpose of this chapter is to explore some examples of how counselling might be used. Each section offers two examples of counselling. One is an example of how not to do it. The second is an example of an improved version. As we have already discovered, there is no right way to counsel. Much depends on the circumstances at the time, the people concerned and a wide range of other variables. On the other hand, it is not difficult to get things wrong, either. The first examples in those below probably try to mimic ordinary conversation too closely. They represent a coming and going of exchanges between the two people without the focus being on either. The point of counselling is to focus almost exclusively on the other person and thus ensure that the conversation is a therapeutic one.

None of these examples is perfect. Read through them and see to what degree you would use the approaches offered. You may find that some of the examples offered as ways of not doing counselling are fine. If so, ask yourself why they have been included. Try to discuss your thoughts with a colleague.

Counselling in general nursing

There are numerous chances to practise counselling skills in general nursing from admitting a person to hospital to helping a relative to face bad news. Also, there are many occasions on which counselling colleagues becomes a priority. Many nurses find that they are faced with emotions that are brought to the surface by the nature of the job. It is very useful if another colleague can help in the talking through of such feelings. Without these opportunities to work through our feelings, we run the risk of bottling them up and this can lead to burnout – emotional and physical exhaustion caused by job-related stress. We no longer have to keep a stiff upper lip. We need to care for each other. Counselling is one method of helping in this way.

How it should not be done

'How is my father getting on?'
'He's fine.'
'Is he getting any better?'
'I think you better ask the doctor about that.'
'But what do you think? You see him every day.'
'He's as well as can be expected.'
'Do you think he will get much better?'
'Well, seeing as what's wrong with him . . . you have to be realistic. I know it's difficult but you have to realize that he's not so young any more. Everyone finds it difficult to accept, I know, but we have to be realistic . . .'
'Does he go to physiotherapy?'
'Sometimes. He's difficult sometimes, though. Because he's not well, he's sometimes a bit crabby. I think that's how older people are, sometimes. I know, my father can get very crabby!'
'I wonder if he would be better off at home.'
'He's being very well looked after, here. Only you can decide if you would be able to look after him at home. I think he's better off here. We can look after him properly, here.'
'But I could look after him at home!'
'I know you think you could, but it would be a dreadful strain. A lot of people think like you. They think that they could manage and then they don't. Then the trouble really starts. As I say, I think we have to be realistic.'

How it might be done

'How is my father getting on?'
'He seems to be more settled now.'
'I'm glad of that. He seemed so anxious when I came last time.'
'How are *you* coping?'
'Some days it's alright. Then I have days when I think I'm never going to get used to him being in hospital.'
'You find it hard going?'

'Yes. These last two days have been particularly difficult. It was alright when my father was first admitted. It was a relief, I suppose. Then, when I had time on my hands, I began to worry about whether or not I had done the right thing. It's difficult to know . . . Do you think I should have him back at home?'
'It may be a bit early to think about that . . .'
'But did I do the right thing? I suppose other people have to accept that they can't cope at home . . .'
'A lot of people do find it difficult . . .'
'And you feel that he is settling down?'
'Yes. He has his moments, but by and large he is settling.'
'He's not perfect, I know. He can be difficult at times.'
'We can cope.'
'Yes, I know you can. Thank you for listening to me. I'm sorry to have gone on at you so much but it makes such a difference when I can talk about some of these things.'
'I don't mind at all. If you want to talk again, we could meet next time you come.'
'Thank you.'

Counselling in nursing education

Tutors and lecturers often have to talk to their students about progress, assessments and other aspects of the educational and training processes. As we noted in the previous chapter, there are two sorts of counselling that may occur in an educational context: educational counselling itself and personal counselling. The examples that follow are those of educational counselling. If you can, read through these examples and discuss both approaches with a colleague. Reflect, too, on the degree to which either is typical of conversations that *you* have had with other people.

How it should not be done

'Hello. Could I talk to you for a few minutes?'
'Yes. Hold on. I'll be right with you. Have we got an appointment?'
'No. Sorry. I just wanted to talk.'
'That's OK. I'll just sign these letters. Carry on. I'm listening. Are you doing alright on the ward?'
'Yes, fine. I'm just a bit worried about my essays.'
'What about them?'
'I don't seem to be improving on my marks.'
'You're passing, aren't you?'
'Yes. I'm passing but I'm not really improving.'
'I wouldn't worry. You pass if you get 95 per cent, you pass if you get 45 per cent. What's the problem?'

'I'd just like to know that I was getting on alright. I read quite a lot but I have problems with my writing.'
'Most people do. My spelling is appalling! As long as you plan your work before you start, you should be OK. You did alright in the last exams, didn't you?'
'Yes.'
'You're doing alright. Your last paper was really interesting.'
'Do you think I'm doing OK, then?'
'Yes, fine.'
'And you don't think I should worry?'
'No. You're bright enough. You should have no problems. Give my regards to David when you get back to the ward and don't forget, if you ever need any help, just let me know.'
'Thanks.'

How it might be done

'Hello. Could I talk to you for a few minutes?'
'Hello Sarah. Of course you can talk. I was expecting you. Sit down.'
'Thanks. It's just that I'm a bit worried about my essays.'
'What seems to be the problem?'
'I don't seem to be improving.'
'Your marks are always about the same?'
'Yes. I am passing and everything. I just don't seem to be getting any better.'
'What do you see as the difficulty?'
'I don't really. I always think that they will be alright.'
'Tell me how you go about writing an essay.'
'Well, I sit down and get the books together, write out some notes, make a few headlines and then write.'
'Do you "brainstorm" your ideas, before you write?'
'No. The ideas usually come to me as I write.'
'Does anyone ever suggest that your writing needs more structure?'
(Laughs). 'Yes, now you say it, they always say that about my papers.'
'So what can you do?'
'I could write more headings.'
'And plan your work in more detail?'
'It seems so boring, though!'
'You want to get better marks and write better essays . . .'
'Yes, I see what you mean.'
'Do you think you can do it?'
'Yes, I know I can.'
'Good! Is anything else worrying you?'
'No. I'm fine. I'm not even worried about my essays, I just wanted to do them better.'
'Fine. See you up on the ward.'
'Thanks. See you soon.'

Counselling in psychiatric nursing

There will be times in psychiatric nursing when patients are offered formal psychotherapy of one of the sorts referred to in the last chapter. Sometimes, though, it will be appropriate to offer counselling. The examples below are drawn from conversations with someone who is suffering from anxiety and illustrate two approaches.

How it should not be done

'What seems to be the problem, mostly?'
'I get a funny feeling in my stomach and I feel very tense.'
'We all get tense at times. I know I do. What do you think has caused it?'
'I don't know. I wasn't like it last week.'
'Perhaps you're worried about something.'
'I suppose so. It doesn't feel very nice, though.'
'What are you going to do about it?'
'I'm not sure. I get a bit panicky sometimes. It feels horrible.'
'Don't you think that everyone feels like that sometimes? It's not abnormal you know.'
'I know, but I just wish I knew what to do about it, that's all.'
'Have you tried taking some deep breaths and trying to slow your breathing rate down a bit? That often helps.'
'I could try that.'
'Do you want to have a go, then?'
'What, now?'
'Yes.'
'OK.' (Takes deep breaths.) 'How long does it take to work?'
'Well you have to allow yourself to slow down quite a lot. Keep at it. I'll come back and see you later on and see how you are.'
'Thank you.'
'And don't forget. Try not to worry so much. You don't need to. We are here to look after you. Nothing bad can happen.'
'OK.'

How it might be done

'What seems to be the problem, mostly?'
'I get a funny feeling in my stomach and I feel very tense.'
'When does this happen?'
'In the evenings, mostly.'
'What, after supper?'
'Later than that – towards bedtime, I suppose.'
'Towards bedtime . . .'

'Well, it sort of creeps up on me during the evening.'
'And then you get to feel tense?'
'Yes, it starts in my stomach and I start to think I'm going to get all panicky.'
'How are you feeling at the moment?'
'I could get like it now.'
'But you're not?'
'No. I'm stopping myself.'
'How are you doing that?'
'By talking and thinking of other things.'
'And that works?'
'Yes.'
'How is it different in the evenings?'
'I don't have too many people to talk to, I suppose.'
'When you talk and think of other things, you don't get so anxious?'
'No. I'm feeling better already – just by talking.'
'We could meet in the evenings, if you would like to, and talk a bit and see what happens.'
'Thank you. I would appreciate that – it really does make a difference.'
'OK. I'll see you again tomorrow at 7 o'clock.'
'Yes. Thanks very much.'

Counselling in the community

There are many different sorts of community nurses, from district nurses to community psychiatric nurses. Also, health visitors play a large role in visiting people in their homes and talking to clients in the community. The obvious difference between the hospital and the community setting is that the community nurse is seeing the client on his or her own territory. This can make the process of counselling easier for the client, but may make it more difficult for the nurse. We all like to work in places that we know. What the community nurse has to do is to learn to adapt quickly to being able to counsel in lots of different settings. Sometimes, too, the seating arrangements may not be ideal. It is helpful, in counselling, to sit opposite the client so that you can see them clearly. People's houses are not necessarily arranged for this to be easily achieved. In many houses, the focal point of the main room is the television. Community nurses, then, may have to compromise.

Increasingly, too, community nurses have to make quick decisions about whether or not to refer a family or a family member on to another caring agency. There has been much coverage in the news about the increase of child abuse. Community nurses have to be tactful in the way that they interpret conversations with children and their parents. They often have to tread a fine line between being overcautious and being careless. Exactly how to tread this line is one of the topics covered in most community nursing courses. However, the community nurse who undertakes counselling in people's homes should also be alert to the content of what she is hearing. It is no longer sufficient merely to see counselling as a means of helping the individual. In community counselling, the 'client' is the whole family.

How it should not be done

'It's good to see you, I've had a horrible week.'
'Why, what's happened.'
'I've just been unable to cope, that's all.'
'What do you mean?'
'Oh, I don't know, really. I keep getting nervous about leaving the house.'
'What, frightened?'
'Not really. I just wonder what would happen if I got stuck in here, that's all.'
'It sounds, to me, as though you're not going out *enough*. Does your husband take you out?'
'No. I wouldn't want him to, either.'
'It might be a good idea. You don't want to get stuck inside four walls all day.'
'No. I do go out. It's just that I get a bit worried, that's all.'
'I suppose everyone has their moments. Try to make a few friends. Talk to your neighbours. I'm sure they feel like that sometimes. Now, how is your leg?'
'Oh. My leg? It's much better. I'll show you.'

How it might be done

'It's good to see you, I've had a horrible week.'
'Do you want to tell me about it?'
'Well, it started with something my husband said. He said that I was getting to look fairly old and untidy. He often says tactless things like that and I didn't mind too much. It's just after that I began to worry.'
'What about?'
'Our relationship and things. We don't seem to get on very well these days. We don't talk to each other. He just comes in and sits in front of the box. I'm not sure that I really *want* to talk to him about anything in particular – I'd just like to know that I could.'
'What *would* you talk to him about, do you think?'

'Oh, I don't know. Silly things. Like I've got a bit nervous that I may be agoraphobic . . . It's silly really.'
'You worry about getting trapped in the house?'
'Yes. It's only because I have no one to talk to.'
'I don't think it's silly. I think I can understand how you feel.'
'I just get so miserable. Once he's gone to work, there's nobody. All the neighbours tend to be out to work and I haven't got a lot of friends in this area.'
'What do you think needs to be done?'
'I need to get out, I suppose. I need to talk to David, as well.'
'Could you do that?'
'Yes, I think so. If I worked at it. Yes, I will do that.'
'I could come back and talk a bit more with you, too, if you wanted.'
'Yes, I would like that. Just talking a bit this afternoon has helped. I know I'm not agoraphobic really, its just that your imagination takes over sometimes, when you don't talk. I know that once I get talking to David again, things will be easier. It's surprising how you can live with someone and never talk to them.'
'I'll see you on Wednesday afternoon, then, at 3.00.'
'Yes, thanks again.'

What are the common factors?

It is possible to draw out of all of the above examples some of the common factors that make counselling effective. As in the previous chapter, for the moment, these are simply listed. In the chapters that follow, each of these issues will be dealt with at some length. See if you can add to the list or see whether or not you would cross some of them out. The common factors are:

- Listening
- Encouraging
- Enabling
- Expression of feelings
- Exploring
- Easing of tension
- Following the client's lead
- Resolution of problems.

Activities for exploring the issues in this chapter

The activities for working with the issues in this chapter are straightforward ones. Mostly, they require observation of other people at work. If, as we have discussed, listening is the most important aspect of counselling, it is vital to begin to enhance your listening straightaway. Therefore, the first two activities encourage you to do just that.

Activity one: listen to nurses talking and compare the conversations that you have read through in this chapter with those that you hear around you. To what degree do you think that nurses are 'good listeners'?

Activity two: begin to practise listening. For the moment, all this entails is that you hold back in conversations. When you would normally say something, resist for a moment or two more and allow the other person to carry on. Learning to listen must be a conscious act. Like all other skills, it takes practice to become a good listener.

Activity three: read more about counselling.

Activity four: begin to identify the sorts of situations in which counselling might help.

Questions for reflection and discussion

- To what degree is counselling used in your field of nursing?
- Who would you say were the most effective counsellors in the health care field?
- Should counselling be an aspect of all types of nursing?

3

Qualities of the counsellor

Nurses and counsellors come in all shapes and sizes. It has been acknowledged in the first chapter that all nurses need counselling skills. Like all skills, though, some will be better at it than others. Much of the time, counselling is dependent not upon a range of particular skills but on the *relationship* that develops between the two people concerned. Also, it helps to be fairly outgoing and open. Clearly, the person who is very withdrawn and insular is unlikely to find themselves being approached as a counsellor. Counselling, by its nature, calls for certain personal qualities and it is these that are discussed in this chapter.

The idea of personal qualities does not mean that we all have to be much the same sort of person to take on a counselling role. One of the problems of some counselling courses that depend heavily on counselling skills is that they can sometimes turn out clones. By this I mean that it is possible to spot some 'professional counsellors' a mile off. They use language in a certain way, they sit in certain positions and they use eye contact in a studied manner. The point, of course, is simply that such behaviour can put people off. Rather than make good counsellors, such behaviour can lessen the chance of other people approaching them as counsellors. In the end, despite the discussion on the qualities of a good counsellor and in spite of the emphasis on developing certain counselling skills, we need to be ourselves. As we shall note towards the end of this chapter, self-awareness can help here. Also, though, we need to lose a certain professional gloss that we sometimes develop as we become nurses. We need to be able to face the other person as a reasonably normal, ordinary human being. We do not have to face them as a professional counsellor, as a superhuman being or as someone who has sorted out all of his or her problems. We need to be natural. Unfortunately, it often takes a long time to learn to be natural!

Personal warmth

Warmth, in the nursing relationship refers to being approachable and open to the patient or colleague. Schulman (1982) argues that the following characteristics are involved in demonstrating the concept of warmth: equal worth, absence of blame, non-defensiveness and closeness. Warmth is as much a frame of mind as a skill and perhaps one developed through being honest with yourself and being prepared to be open with others It also involves treating the other person as an equal human being.

Martin Buber (1958) the philosopher and therapist made a distinction between the 'I–it' relationship and the 'I–Thou' (or 'I–you') relationship. In the I–it relationship, one person treats the other as an object. In the I–thou relationship, there occurs a meeting of persons, transcending any differences there may be in terms of status, background, lifestyle, belief or value systems. In the I–thou relationship there is a sense sharing and of mutuality, a sense that can be contagious and is of particular value in nursing.

Unfortunately, it is all too easy to turn patients into objects in the way suggested by Buber. Consider, for example the nurse who refers to the 'appendix in bed 5'. In talking in this way, he or she is treating that patient not as a thinking and feeling person but as an object – an 'appendix'. After all, it is not the appendix that is in bed 5 but the person who has had his appendix removed!

There is an interesting point that needs to be discussed here. While warmth must be offered by the nurse to the client, the feeling may not necessarily be reciprocated by the client. There is, as well, another problem with the notion of warmth. We all perceive personal qualities in different sorts of ways. One person's warmth is another person's sickliness or sentimentality. We cannot guarantee how our warmth will be perceived by the other person. In a more general way, however, warmth may be compared to coldness. It is clear that the cold person would not be the ideal person to undertake helping another person in a nursing setting! It is salutary, however, to reflect on the degree to which there are cold people working in the nursing arena and to question why this may be so. It is possible that interpersonal skills training may help this situation, for it may be that some cold people are unaware of their coldness.

To a degree, however, our relationships with others tend to be self-monitoring. We anticipate, as we go on with a relationship, the effect we are having on others and modify our presentation of self accordingly. Thus we soon get to know if our warmth is too much for the patient or colleague or is being perceived by him in a negative way. This ability constantly to monitor ourselves and our relationships is an important part of the process of developing interpersonal and counselling skills.

I believe that it is not difficult to appreciate that some people clearly are perceived by lots of other people as warm while others are perceived as cold. By way of testing this out, think about your own colleagues and friends and try, if you can, to divide them into warm or cold. No doubt some will fall through the middle of this divide and be uncategorizable!

Genuineness

Genuineness, too, is another important aspect of the counselling relationship. In one sense, the issue is black or white. We either genuinely care for the person in front of us or we do not. We cannot easily fake professional interest. We must be interested. Some people, however, will interest us more than others. Often, those clients who remind us of our own problems or our own personalities will interest us most of all. This is not so important as our having a genuine interest in the fact that the relationship is happening at all.

On the surface of it, there may appear to be a conflict between the concept of genuineness and the self-monitoring alluded to above. Self-monitoring may be thought of as 'artificial' or contrived and therefore not genuine. The genuineness discussed here relates to the nursing professional's interest in the human relationship that is developing between the two people. Any ways in which that relationship can be enhanced must serve a valuable purpose. It is quite possible to be genuine and yet aware of what is happening: genuine and yet committed to increasing interpersonal competence.

Empathy

The term empathy is usually used to convey the idea of the ability to enter the perceptual world of the other person: to see the world as they see it. It also suggests an ability to convey this perception to the other person. Kalisch (1971) defines empathy as the 'ability to perceive accurately the feelings of another person and to communicate this understanding to him'.

Empathy is different to sympathy. Sympathy suggests feeling sorry for the other person or, perhaps, identifying with how they feel. If a person sympathizes, they imagine themselves as being in the other person's position. With empathy the person tries to imagine how it is to be the other person. Feeling sorry for that person does not really come into it.

The process of developing empathy involves something of an act of faith. When we empathize with another person, we cannot know what the outcome of that empathizing will be. If we pre-empt the outcome of our empathizing, we are already not empathizing – we are thinking of solutions and of ways of influencing the client towards a particular goal that we have in mind. The process of empathizing involves entering into the perceptual world of the other person without necessarily knowing where that process will lead.

Developing empathic understanding is the process of exploring the client's world, with the client, neither judging nor necessarily offering advice. Perhaps it can be achieved best through the process of carefully attending and listening to the other person and, perhaps, by use of the skill known as 'reflection', which is discussed in a later chapter of this book. It is also a way of being, a disposition towards the client, a willingness to explore the other person's problems and to allow the other person to express themselves fully. Again, as with all aspects of the client-centred approach to caring, the empathic approach is underpinned by the idea that it is the client, in the end, who will find her own way through and will find her own answers to her problems in living. To be empathic is to be a fellow traveller, a friend to the person as they undertake the search. Empathic understanding, then, invokes the notion of befriending.

There are limitations to the degree to which we can truly empathize. Because we all live in different worlds based on our particular culture, education, physiology, belief systems and so forth, we all view that world slightly differently. Thus, to empathize truly with another person would involve actually becoming that other person! We can, however, strive to get as close to the perceptual world of the other by listening and attending and by suspending judgement. We can also learn to forget ourselves, temporarily, and give ourselves as completely as we can to the other person. There is an interesting paradox involved here. First, we need self-awareness to enable us to develop empathy. Then we need to forget ourselves in order truly to give our empathic attention to the other person.

Gerard Egan (1990) offers a useful summary of the way in which empathy can be useful in the counselling or helping relationship. He suggests that empathy can:

- Build the relationship
- Stimulate self-exploration
- Check understandings
- Provide support
- Lubricate communication
- Focus attention
- Restrain the helper
- Pave the way

Unconditional positive regard

Carl Rogers phrase 'unconditional positive regard' (Rogers, 1967), conveys a particularly important predisposition towards the client, by the nurse. Rogers also called it 'prizing' or even just 'accepting'. It means that the client is viewed with the dignity and valued as a worthwhile and positive human being. The 'unconditional' prefix refers to the idea that such regard is offered without any preconditions. Often in relationships, some sort of reciprocity is demanded: I will like you (or love you) so long as you return that liking or loving. Rogers is asking that the feelings that the nursing professional holds for the client should be undemanding and not requiring reciprocation.

There is a suggestion of an inherent goodness within the client, bound up in Rogers' notion of unconditional positive regard. This notion of persons as essentially good can be traced back, at least to Rousseau's 'Emile' and is philosophically problematic. Arguably, notions such as goodness and badness are social constructions and to argue that a person is born good or bad is fraught. However, as a practical starting point in the nursing relationship, it seems to be a good idea that we assume an inherent, positive and life-asserting characteristic in the client. It seems difficult to argue otherwise. It would be odd, for instance, to engage in the process of counselling with the view that the person was essentially bad, negative and unlikely to grow or develop!

Unconditional positive regard, then, involves a deep and positive feeling for the other person, perhaps equivalent, in the health professions to what Alistair Campbell has called 'moderated love' (Campbell, 1984). He talks of 'lovers and professors', suggesting that certain professionals profess to love, thus claiming both the ability to be professional and to express altruistic love or disinterested love for others. It is interesting that Campbell seems to be suggesting that a nursing professional can professionally care or even professionally love her client.

Can we offer our patients unconditional positive regard? Sometimes, it seems like the counsel of perfection. Few of us would be able to sustain it with every person we met. Few of us would probably be able to sustain it with any one person all of the time. Perhaps, in the end, it is a goal to aim at – an ideal. I can think of plenty of people whom I have counselled for whom I have felt nothing like this sort of regard! On the other hand, I suspect that the best counselling and most useful counselling always occur when the counsellor *is* accepting of the other person – warts and all.

Intuition

Intuition is perhaps the most undervalued of personal qualities. Intuition refers to knowledge and insight that arrives independently of the senses. In other words we just know. Ornstein (1975) who studies the literature on the differences between the two sides of the brain identified intuition with the right side. He argued that the two sides have qualitatively different functions. The left side is concerned with cognitive processes and with rationality. The right is more to do with holism, creativity and intuition, according to Ornstein. If he is right, the implication is that if the intuitive aspect is developed further (along with creativity) then both sides of the brain will function optimally. Ornstein argues that the present Western culture is dominated by the left brain approach to education and development. He calls for an education system that honours creativity and intuition *alongside* the development of rationality.

Perhaps we neglect intuition through fear of it or concern that it may not be trusted. On the other hand, it is likely that we all have hunches that when followed turn out to be right. Many aspects of nursing require the nurse to be intuitive. Sometimes, in order to empathize with another person we have to guess at what they are feeling. Sometimes we seem to know what they are feeling. Certainly, counselling depends to a fair degree on this intuitive ability. Carl Rogers, founder of client-centred counselling noted that when he had a hunch about something that was happening in a counselling session, it invariably helped if he verbalized that intuition (Rogers, 1967). Using intuition consciously and openly takes courage and sometimes it is wrong. However, used hand in hand with more traditional forms of thinking, it can enhance the nurse/patient relationship in a way that logic, on its own, never can.

Caring

In order really to help clients in counselling, we must care for them. Now, this may sound obvious, after all, we belong to a caring profession. But what does it mean to care? Milton Mayeroff, in an important analysis of the meaning of caring in human relationships (Mayeroff, 1971), describes caring as a process which offers people (both the carer and the cared for individual), opportunities for personal growth.

Major aspects of caring in the analysis include: knowledge, alternating rhythms (learning from experience), patience, honesty, trust, humility, hope, and courage. These elements are discussed in more detail here, although the discussion is a little different to the one that Mayeroff offers.

Knowledge

In order to care for someone, we must know certain things. First, we must know who they are. Think of a friendship. Friendships develop because as we learn more about the other person, we acknowledge that we like what we get to know. If we did not like it, the friendship would not develop at all. In the context of nursing, we must also get to know the patient in order to care for them.

In another sense, however, we need knowledge to *use* and to give to the patient. In the sense of knowledge to use, we need to know certain things about what is wrong with the other person in order to help him or her. Thus, in caring for a person with diabetes, we need to know various things about the nature of the condition.

It is worth noting, however, that there are definite limits to what we need know in order to care for others. We cannot know very much about what is best for the other person when it comes to his personal or emotional life. It is tempting, when someone has personal problems to offer advice. Such advice is only rarely helpful. One moment's reflection will reveal the fact that each of us lives a very different personal life to the next person. While as nurses we can all come to know something about the nature of diabetes, we cannot come to know very much about the personal life of the patient. When it comes to personal and emotional issues, the patient is the expert on his own situation. Caring, here, consists of *resisting* the temptation to tell the patient how to live his life or how to sort out his emotional problems.

Alternating rhythms

Consider any relationship that you have with another person, whether in the family, with friends or with colleagues. In all these different situations, the *intensity* of the relationship fluctuates. Sometimes we feel very close to the other person, sometimes we feel quite distant. According to Mayeroff, this is an example of the 'alternating rhythms' of any caring relationship. No relationship (and that includes one with a patient) can stay intense and close for any length of time. There seems to be a natural cycle in the caring relationship – what may be described as its waxing and waning.

There is another sense of the term 'alternating rhythms'. This is the idea that we may have to modify continuously the ways in which we react with another person. Sometimes, one approach works. On another occasion, another is required. People vary from day to day. What works with them one day does not necessarily work with them on another. T. S. Eliot once wrote that we 'die to each other daily' (Eliot, 1965). That is to say that since we last saw some one, lots of things have happened to them: they have changed and become other than they were.

If this is the case, then each new meeting with a person involves us *reknowing* them with meeting them afresh. Thus, in the context of caring, we must learn this process of remeeting and reknowing the person for whom we care.

Patience

Caring for another person involves taking your time. While we may hope that a relationship could warm up quickly, very often other people take time to get to know us and to allow us to care for them. Again, think of a close emotional relationship that you have with a friend. That relationship did not come about overnight. It took time for both of you to get to know each other and get to like each other. In this sense, then, the caring relationship requires patience. Caring relationships, whether with friends or with patients, cannot be rushed.

In another sense, too, patience requires tolerance. We need to appreciate that other people are not the same as us. We are required, therefore to accept the person for whom we are caring, warts and all. We cannot hope that the other person will come to be like us. Such a position requires patience: both with the other person and with ourselves.

Honesty

Honesty is not simply a question of not doing things like telling lies or deceiving the other person, but involves being open to sharing with them exactly how we feel. It involves being able to tell them the truth, whether that truth consists of factual information that they need, or whether it is concerned with our feelings for them. A prerequisite for being able to be honest with other people is being able to be honest with ourselves. A necessary requirement for being honest with others, then, is a degree of self-awareness, of being able honestly to appraise our own thoughts, feelings, beliefs and values. Put simply, if we do not know certain things about ourselves, we do not know that we do not know them!

All this is trickier than it first seems. It is quite difficult being honest with yourself and then, sometimes it seems almost impossible to be honest with others. You may have often found yourself thinking, 'I'll tell him exactly how I feel', only to find yourself *saying* something different. We use all sorts of complicated mental processes to protect ourselves. One of them is avoiding being honest. Yet this is one quality we must *try* to develop if we are to expect people in counselling to be honest with us.

Trust

Trust is a clear requirement for caring. Just as we learn to allow a child to find things out for himself and to make mistakes for himself, so, with adults we must be able to trust them to learn from their own experience, to make decisions for themselves and so forth. It is easy for us, as nurses, to become compulsive carers: we smother the people for whom we are caring because we cannot trust them to take care of themselves. Trust, then, also involves letting go. It involves an element of risk taking and accepting that other people find things out in their own way and live their lives differently from us. Often, mistrust in other people demonstrates a distrust of ourselves. We trust others more when we are secure in ourselves. Thus, again, the need for self-awareness and self-exploration.

Humility

To care for another person is a great honour. If another person trusts herself to us, we need to be aware of the great responsibility that this involves. We cannot afford to become too flattered by the other person turning to us for care. We need to stay humble and to appreciate our own inadequacies and limitations.

If we are not humble, we are likely to feel an overvalued sense of our own knowledge and views. To be humble, however, suggests that we have much more to learn. In the caring relationship, if we stay humble we stay open to new learning and to finding out more about the other person. Also, we need to remain humble about the degree to which we can help people at all. Counselling does not offer all the answers and we must be reserved about our successes. The true test of counselling is whether or not the client does anything as a result of our counselling. The talking part is easy: it is the changing that is difficult.

Hope

To care for another person is to affirm that we believe in his ability to overcome problems and adversity. We cannot care without hope. If we do, we may just as well abandon the whole enterprise, for why are we bothering to care at all?

To counsel at all, suggests hope. As we grow fond of someone (which is often, though not always, the outcome of caring) we want to know them more and expect to see more of them. If we do not have hope, then we cannot expect this desire to be fulfilled. In the end, we would not enter into a counselling relationship if we really thought that we had no hope, either for ourselves or for the person with whom we were counselling.

Courage

A lot is at stake when we care for someone else. Despite our efforts, despite our hope, they may not recover or, less dramatically, they may not care for us. They may not even like us! Thus to care is something of a gamble. Just as we cannot know the future, we cannot anticipate the outcome of our caring. Thus to care takes considerable courage.

It takes courage, too, to share ourselves with another person. While caring may not always be a reciprocal relationship, it is likely that we will need to give of ourselves in the caring role. We may also need to tell the person for whom we are caring things about ourselves. As you tell me about you, the unwritten rule is that I tell you about me.

In this sense, caring is a process of coming to know the other person. This sharing of self takes courage. we are all vulnerable and all fear that our self-disclosure may not be accepted by the other person. Usually, of course, it is. There are occasions when it will not be. It is for such occasions that we need to have a reserve of courage.

These, then, are some of the elements involved in caring for another person. It is not an exhaustive account. Suffice to say, though, that unless we care for the client, we are unlikely to be very successful in our counselling.

Sense of humour

Humour plays a part in most people's lives. While it is not an immediately obvious quality for the counselling, I believe that it is an important one. Humour has an almost universal power to defuse tension, relieve stress and bring a sense of perspective to a situation. It is as though if we can laugh at ourselves, we get a view of the real size of the problem. Helping people to laugh gently at themselves can be therapeutic. That is not to say that the counsellor should in any way be fatuous, ridiculing or sarcastic – far from it. Suffice to say that small doses of gentle humour can make all the difference to effective counselling. On the other hand, the counsellor who is too earnest and humourless is one who can often appear inhuman and of no real value to the client. The psychologist, Carl Jung, once noted that the person who has lost his or her sense of humour has lost an important aspect of their spiritual make up.

Arnold and Boggs (1989) note the following variables that contribute to the successful use of humour as a communication strategy:

- Knowledge of the client's response pattern
- An overly intense situation
- Timing
- The client's developmental level.

In other words, we need to know something about the client's *own* sense of humour, we can use humour to take the sting out of a situation, we need to time our use of humour carefully and we need to be aware of the client's ability to appreciate our use of humour. As Synder (1985) noted, many studies have noted how idiosyncratic humour is: what I find funny, you may not.

A sense of the tragic

This is almost the opposite pole of the previous quality. All counsellors need to be acutely aware of people's ability to experience tragedy. The Buddhist faith notes one central truth: that all life is suffering. The sense of the tragic is an acknowledgement of the tragic aspects of life: the unreasonableness of much of what happens to us, the arbitrariness of much of life and so on. Without a sense of the tragic and of other people's ability to experience tragedy, we are likely to take only a superficial view of other people's suffering. This can produce stilted and unhelpful responses such as 'Don't worry. I'm sure its not as bad as you think. It'll all work out in the end.'

A balance between, on the one hand, having a sense of humour and, on the other, having a profound sense of the tragic is an ideal one for the counsellor. In a sense, the two are complementary, for, almost paradoxically, both contain elements of the other. The most tragic situation can have humorous elements to it: some humour is also tragic.

Self-awareness

Self-awareness is the process of getting to know yourself better. It is a vital quality in counselling for the following reasons:

- It helps you to avoid confusing your problems with the client's problems. Without awareness, it is often easy to confuse our 'ego boundaries' with those of the other person. That is to say that it is easy to lose sight of what we think and what the other person thinks. As an example of how this happens, try to recall when you were under the influence of someone who had a stronger personality than you. When this happened, it was probably difficult to know whether some of the things you thought were your thoughts or the thoughts of the other person. Without clear ego boundaries, we are often easily influenced by what others say and lose sight of ourselves.
- It allows you to work through periods of personal stress. Self-awareness helps you to appreciate and understand your limits.
- It allows you to work intentionally. That is to say, self-awareness can help you to choose what you say and do in the counselling relationship rather than just allowing it to happen. With awareness, we choose: without it, we are not even aware of the choices we have.

Much has been written about self-awareness elsewhere and you may find *Learning Human Skills* (Burnard, 1990) useful as an introduction to the topic. Suffice to say, here, that getting to know more about your own thoughts, feelings and behaviour is a worthwhile enterprise for all nurses and a vital one for anyone who wants to work in any sort of counselling.

What, though, can a person become aware of? Here is a shortlist of some of the issues that you can work on:

- Beliefs
- Values
- Prejudices
- Likes and dislikes
- How others see you
- Your view of yourself
- Religious beliefs or lack of them

- Political beliefs
- Sexual preferences
- Fears and anxieties
- Knowledge
- Skills
- Strengths
- Deficits.

Developing personal qualities: a checklist

In order to being to focus on self-awareness, here is a list of questions for you to consider. Work through the list, considering your answers to each question. Then consider what it might be like to reverse your answer. In other words, try to imagine what it would be like to hold exactly the opposite beliefs, views and so on, to the ones that you hold at the moment. This process of working with opposites is both helpful in developing self-awareness and also often useful in counselling. For example, it can be helpful to invite the client to express the opposite of what they are saying when they seem half-hearted in a particular response. Here is one example of the use of opposites used in this way.

> 'Of course, if my daughter *did* leave home, it wouldn't worry me very much . . .'
> 'Can you try saying the opposite of that?'
> 'What do you mean . . . ? If my daughter left home it *would* worry me a great deal. Oh! I see what you mean . . . yes, I think it would worry me . . .'

Below are the questions to consider. If you can, work through them on your own and then share your answers with a colleague. In this way you can begin to see the degree to which you are like other people and the ways in which you are different from them. Again, such differences are important and can help you to appreciate just how different and how similar we can be. A triplet attributed to Gordon Allport is useful here. He is said to have suggested that:

Everyone is in some ways like:
1 No other person
2 Some other people
3 All other people

Self-Awareness questions

- Are you happy with life?
- Are you responsible for everything that you do?
- Are you a cautious person?
- Are you happy with your job or your course?
- Are you careful about what you eat?
- Could you imagine being a conscientious objector?
- Do you think that people do not know the 'real' you?'
- Do you think that you are attractive?
- Do you think that abortion should be available on demand?
- Do you lose your temper easily?
- Do you mind if people ask you what you earn?
- Do you think that we are also responsible for other people?
- Do you believe in God?
- Do you think that you have changed very much over the past five years?
- Do you think that people should talk freely about sex?
- Do you think that you are intelligent?
- Do you think that people are responsible for themselves?
- Do you consider yourself British or European?
- Do you have a sense of humour?
- Do you watch 'soaps' on the television?
- Do you think that people watch too much television?
- Do you think that the prison system is a good one?
- Generally speaking, do you like other people?
- Have you ever broken the law?
- Have you travelled widely?
- How would you react if you found out that you were HIV positive?
- How would you like to change your appearance?
- If you could live anywhere, where would you choose to live?
- If you could travel anywhere in the world, where would you go?
- If you were to change sex, what sort of man or woman would you be?
- In what ways do you need to change more?
- Of all the people that you know, who is the most important?
- Should gay people be allowed to 'marry'?
- What do you like least about yourself?
- What is the worst thing that could happen to you?
- What is the best thing about you?

- What is it about people that you don't like?
- What are the things that you like most about people?
- What do you like most about yourself?
- What are the things that you like least about people?
- What is the worst thing about you?
- What is it about you that has stayed the same?
- What would you most like to change about the world?
- What is the most difficult thing about working with other people?
- What sort of work would you do if you did not work with people?
- What political views do you hold?
- What is the most difficult thing you have ever had to do?
- What *wouldn't* you talk about to other people?
- Who would you most like to get to know better?
- Who are you most afraid of?
- Who is the person that you know that is most different to you?
- Who is the person that you know that is most like you?
- Would you say that you were an optimist?
- Would you say that you were broad minded?

Requirements for effective counselling

This chapter has explored a variety of personal qualities that are necessary for a person to practise as an effective counsellor. Before moving on to examine the model of counselling that is being recommended, it is important to recap and to bring together those factors that a person needs in order to function as a counsellor. Table 3.1 offers examples of the requirements a person might need, examples of those requirements and methods by which they may be learned. In the end, they turn out to be a mix of both formally learned aspects and those that are less formally learned – through the process of living, itself.

Activity for developing the qualities

Activity one: read through this chapter and think about the qualities described in it. Then, consider the degree to which these qualities apply to:

Table 3.1 Requirements for effective counselling

Requirements for effective counselling	*Examples*	*Learning methods*
Personal qualities	Warmth, sense of humour, genuineness etc	Life experience
Specific counselling skills	Questioning, reflecting, checking, etc	Formal training, practice
Life experience	Home life, work, relationships, etc	Passage through life
Knowledge base	Psychological theory, sociological theory etc	Reading, formal teaching and learning
Understanding of self and others	Self-awareness, cultural and social awareness	Introspection, observation of others, sensitivity

- Someone you identify as an effective counsellor
- Someone you know who is not particularly interpersonally skilled
- One of your parents
- You.

Questions for reflection and discussion

- To what degree are Rogers' qualities of the counsellor idealistic?
- Do you have these qualities and in what measure?
- In your experience, are some people better at counselling than others? If so, what *sort* of people?

4

Types of counselling

Over the past few years many sorts of counselling have been discussed in the literature. Perhaps the sort that has been discussed more than most is the client-centred approach. This chapter reviews some of the approaches and focuses particularly on the client-centred approach, although its limitations are noted and other sorts of counselling are also discussed. In a nursing context, the client-centred approach offers one of the most straightforward approaches to counselling and is the least invasive. Like everything, it does have its limitations, as we shall see.

Client-centred counselling

Client-centred counselling is probably the most widely known type of counselling and possibly the most widely used. The term 'client-centred', first used by Carl Rogers (1951), refers to the notion that it is the client, himself, who is best able to decide how to find the solutions to his problems in living. Client-centred, in this sense may be contrasted with the idea of 'counsellor-centred' or 'professional-centred', both of which may suggest that someone other than the client is the 'expert'. While this may be true when applied to certain concrete factual problems – housing, surgery, legal problems and so forth – it is difficult to see how it can apply to personal life issues. In such cases, it is the client who identifies the problem and the client who, given time and space, can find her way through the problem to the solution.

Murgatroyd (1985) summarizes the client-centred position as follows:

- A person in need has come to you for help
- In order to be helped they need to know that you have understood how they think and feel

- They also need to know that, whatever your own feelings about who or what they are or about what they have or have not done, you accept them as they are
- You accept their right to decide their own lives for themselves
- In the light of this knowledge about your acceptance and understanding of them they will begin to open themselves to the possibility of change and development
- But if they feel that their association with you is conditional upon them changing, they may feel pressurized and reject your help.

The first issues identified by Murgatroyd, the fact of the client coming for help and needing to be understood and accepted, have been discussed in previous chapters. What we need to consider now are ways of helping the person to express themselves, to open themselves and thus to being to change. It is worth noting too, the almost paradoxical nature of Murgatroyd's last point; that if the client feels that their association with you is conditional upon them changing, they may reject your help. Thus we enter into the counselling relationship without even being desirous of the other person changing!

In a sense, this is an impossible state of affairs. If we did not hope for change, we presumably would not enter into the task of counselling in the first place! On another level, however, the point is a very important one. People change at their own rate and in their own time. The process cannot be rushed and we cannot will another person to change. Nor can we expect them to change to become more the sort of person that we would like them to be. We must meet them on their own terms and observe change as they wish and will it to be (or not, as the case may be). This sort of counselling, then, is very altruistic. It demands of us that we make no demands of others.

Client-centred counselling is a process rather than a particular set of skills. It evolves through the relationship that the counsellor has with the client and vice versa. In a sense, it is a period of growth for both parties, for both learn from the other. It also involves the exercise of restraint. The counsellor must restrain herself from offering advice and from the temptation to put the client's life right for him. The outcome of such counselling cannot be predicted nor can concrete goals be set (unless they are devised by the client, at his request). In essence, client-centred counselling involves an act of faith: a belief in the other person's ability to find solutions through the process of therapeutic conversation and through the act of being engaged in a close relationship with another human being.

Certain basic client-centred skills may be identified, although as we have noted, it is the total relationship that is important. Skills exercised in isolation amount to little; the warmth, genuiness and positive regard must also be present. On the other hand, if basic skills are not considered, then the counselling process will probably be shapeless or it will degenerate into the counsellor becoming prescriptive. The skill of standing back and allowing the client to find his own way is a difficult one to learn.

We may well find that the client-centred approach to counselling is linked to a particular period of history – the middle of the 20th century. What characterizes the client-centred approach more than anything is the emphasis on the idea that the client is necessarily the person to sort out his or her own problems. Autonomy and freedom to choose are hallmarks of this approach.

A little reflection, however, will highlight a snag. Put simply, it is this – most of us, for most of the time, do not make autonomous decisions. We do in the literal sense – no one ever can choose for me. But almost all of our decisions are made in a social or relationship context. If I think about most of the important decisions that I make, I do not make them alone. Instead, I consult my wife, children, colleagues and friends. I very rarely just make a decision. I suspect that this is true for very many people. Consider, for example, the following decisions. Accepting, as we have, that only you can make the final decision, consider who else would normally contribute to the decision-making process:

- You need to make a decision about whether or not to buy a house or flat
- You need to decide whether or not to stay in a relationship with someone
- You need to decide whether or not to buy a new car
- You must decide whether or not to stay in nursing.

Sometimes, too, decisions are difficult to make on your own because you do not have enough information to make them. For example, before I knew anything about computers (and wanted to buy one) it was not a simple matter of going out and choosing one. I had to seek the advice of those who knew about computers. Admittedly, I had to decide in the end but the process was made easier by being able to call on the advice of others.

I suspect that nurses and other health professionals may be guilty of overstating the autonomy of the people for whom they care. Most patients and clients, like the rest of us, work and live with a great number of other people. These others all impinge on how and what we decide to do in our lives. Therefore, it is important to consider whether or not the client-centred approach to counselling is always appropriate.

Directive counselling

Directive counselling is the exact opposite to the client-centred approach. It is the process of making suggestions or offering advice to the other person. It is notable that it has tended to be frowned upon in counselling for the past two decades or so. In a study of nurses' attitudes towards counselling, we found that many nurses see their counselling role as a directive one (Morrison and Burnard, 1991). Perhaps, sometimes, it is easier to offer people advice and to make suggestions. Sometimes and in some contexts, it is appropriate. Consider, for example, how odd it would be if the client-centred approach was used by an estate agent:

> 'Good morning. I would like to buy a house and I'm not sure how to go about it.'
> 'What do *you* feel you ought to do about buying a house?

Clearly, the approach does not fit in this situation. In counselling people with life difficulties or emotional problems, however, it is usually much more appropriate to remain in the client-centred mode. As we have often noted, it is the client who is the expert on his or her life. There are times, though, when the directive approach is appropriate. Sometimes, people need specific and accurate advice and help. A short list of times when this may be the case, is as follows:

- The gay person who is anxious to avoid contracting AIDS
- The person who is considering an abortion
- The newly diagnosed diabetic.

While most of these situations could be handled in a client-centred way, it is sometimes more useful to offer direct and clear information. This then allows the other person to make decisions from a position of being informed.

The danger of the directive approach is when it becomes intrusive. It is easy to begin to take over the other person and to try to help him through giving lots of advice and suggestions. Consider, for example, the following exchanges, where a nurse is taking a directive role in counselling. Consider the pros and cons of this method of conducting counselling and think about whether or not a more client-centred approach would be more helpful.

'I feel anxious a lot of the time. I'm not sure why. I suppose I just have to put up with it.'
'It sounds as though you are over-reacting. Lots of people of your age get anxious and it sounds as though you are making too much of it.'
'I suppose so. I do tend to look at things a bit closely.'
'It doesn't help much to become too self-critical. It is sometimes better to take things as they come. Perhaps you need to get out a bit more. I bet you tend to stay at home in the evenings . . . don't you?'
'Not really. I go out about three evenings a week. I just get anxious, that's all.
'It may be something that disappears with time. Perhaps your parents were anxious and that rubbed off on you a bit.'
'My mother was. I'm not sure about my father. I don't think he was a great worrier.'
'You don't *know* that he didn't worry, though, do you?'
'No. I suppose not.'

In this conversation, the main thrust of it is not on how the client feels but on the theories that the counsellor develops about the person being counselled. We are all very good at dreaming up reasons why other people do things but mostly they are fairly wide of the mark. Often, they say more about us than they do about the other person. Consider the above session carried out from a client-centred point of view and notice the differences in outcome – particularly from the point of view of the client.

'I feel anxious a lot of the time. I'm not sure why. I suppose I just have to put up with it.'
'Tell me what happens when you get anxious . . .'
'It just creeps over me, that's all. It starts in my stomach and then seems to take over . . . It's worse in the evenings, when I get home from work.'
'It's worse in the evenings . . .'
'Much worse. I think it must . . . I think it's something to do with my parents . . .'
'What do you think that is?'
'I think I get angry with them but can't tell them. They always want me to do things *their* way.'
'And that upsets you?'

'It upsets me, but I can't tell them. Instead, I get all stewed up and then I get anxious. It sounds silly, but I get nervous that I *will* tell them what I think of them and that makes me more nervous. Perhaps I *should* tell them how I feel.'
'You think you ought to tell them that they upset you?'
'Yes but it wouldn't be easy. That's what I've got to do, though . . .'

Here, the focus is much more on the client's perception of what is going on. The counsellor stays in the background and merely helps the client to verbalize what is going on. No attempt is made to offer advice or make suggestions about what is wrong.

Perhaps the ideal is to be able to work appropriately in both the client-centred and directive modes. One framework for using this balanced approach is Six Category Intervention Analysis (Heron, 1989). The analysis is not a particular theory of counselling nor even a specific type of counselling. It does, however, identify a whole range of possible counselling interventions. It is to this analysis that we now turn.

Client-centred and directive: six category intervention analysis

The six categories in Heron's (1989) analysis are: prescriptive (offering advice); informative (offering information); confronting (challenging); cathartic (enabling the expression of pent-up emotions); catalytic (drawing out); and supportive (confirming or encouraging). The word 'intervention' is used to describe any statement that the counsellor may use. The work 'category' is used to denote a range of related interventions.

Heron calls the first three categories of intervention, (prescriptive, informative and confronting) authoritative and suggests that in using these categories the nurse retains control over the relationship. He calls the second three categories of intervention (cathartic, catalytic and supportive), facilitative and suggests that these enable the client to retain control over the relationship. In other words, the first three are nurse-centred and the second three are client-centred. Another way of describing the difference between the first and second sets of three categories is that the first three are 'You tell me' interventions and the second three are 'I tell you' interventions.

What, then, is the value of such an analysis of therapeutic interventions? First, it identifies the *range* of possible interventions available to the nurse/counsellor. Very often, in day-to-day interactions with others, we stick to repetitive forms of conversation and response simply because we are not aware that the other options are available to us. This analysis identifies an exhaustive range of types of human interventions. Second, by identifying the sorts of interventions we can use, we can act more precisely and with a greater sense of intention. The nurse/patient relationship thus becomes more particular and less haphazard: we know *what* we are saying and also *how* we are saying it. We have greater interpersonal choice.

Third, the analysis offers an instrument for training. Once the categories have been identified, they can be used for students and others to identify their weaknesses and strengths across the interpersonal spectrum. Nurses can, in this way, develop a wide and comprehensive range of interpersonal skills. Heron's six category analysis has been adopted widely in nursing colleges as the means of training people to develop their interpersonal skills.

In two research studies, we invited both student nurses and trained nursing staff to identify their own strengths and weaknesses in terms of the six category intervention analysis (Burnard and Morrison, 1988; Morrison and Burnard, 1989). In the first study, using a convenience sample of 92 trained nurses, these nurses were asked to rank order the six categories according to how skilful they thought they were in using them. Generally speaking, the nurses perceived themselves to be more skilled in using the authoritative categories and less skilled in using the facilitative categories. Having said that, *most* of the nurses perceived themselves as being particularly weak in using *cathartic* and *catalytic* interventions. Overall, they perceived themselves as being best at being supportive.

There were marked similarities in the findings of the second study in which we invited 84 student nurses to rank order the six categories in terms of their perceived strengths and weaknesses in using them. Again, we found an overall picture of greater perceived skill in using authoritative interventions rather than facilitative ones. Students also thought that they were generally most effective in using supportive interventions and not so good at using cathartic and confronting interventions. In general, the results of both studies support Heron's (1989) assertion that a wide range of nurses in our society show a much greater deficit in the skilful use of facilitative interventions than they do in the skilful use of authoritative ones.

These findings suggest that there is still much to be done to help nurses to be more client-centred. They appear to be quite good at being authoritative and advice-giving. If they are to be good all-rounders in the field of counselling, it seems to be important to develop the catalytic, confronting and cathartic elements of Heron's analysis.

Which should I use?

In the last two decades, the accent, in counselling, has tended to be on the client-centred sort. The prevailing wisdom has it that most counsellors should listen to their clients, encourage them to identify their own problems and seek their own solutions. On the other hand, as we have seen, there are occasions in nursing and in medicine, where advice and prescription are necessary. The nurse is likely to be most skilled if she is able to move freely and appropriately between both types of counselling. Unfortunately, though, this can sometimes mean that the slide is towards the more authoritative and nurse-centred sort of counselling. It would appear that, given the choice, nurses tend towards being prescriptive rather than facilitative.

No doubt there are many reasons for this. Nurse training, until fairly recently, has tended to be prescriptive, so it is hardly surprising that nurses, themselves, become prescriptive. Also, nursing is a highly practical profession which aims at problem resolution. It may, at times, seem easier to offer advice as a means of finding quick solutions to difficult problems. Finally, in this short list of possibilities, many nurses are taught to observe patients for signs and symptoms and then to act on what they observe. This is quite different to the client-centred approach to counselling. In this sort of counselling, the nurse is required to get to know the patient as the patient sees him or herself. The nurse is not required merely to observe, report and act. She must get to know the patient from the patient's point of view. This means a considerable change of direction. However, if nursing practice is to develop and grow, it is a change that is worth making.

Levels of counselling

One important aspect of the counselling relationship as it is described in this book is that it is suggested that counselling can work at three levels: feeling level; thinking level; level and concrete level.

People seem to be able to view the world and their problems at these three levels. The feeling level refers to how people feel about what is happening. The thinking level refers to the theories that people have about what is happening. The concrete level refers to what actually happens. Consider, for example, these three snippets of conversation: all refer to the same situation but all three consider that situation from different points of view.

> 'I feel very uncomfortable at home, at the moment' (feeling level).
> 'I think that we all tend to hold onto our feelings about each other in our house' (thinking level).
> 'When I am at home, there are always arguments between me and my parents' (concrete level).

The skilled nurse-counsellor can learn to switch between these levels.

It would seem, too, that some people are predominantly feeling oriented, others tend to focus on thoughts, while others view the world as a series of actual incidences. It is useful, if this is spotted in a particular person, to encourage them to switch levels. These processes and ideas are developed further in later chapters. For the moment, though, read through the following passages and try to identify whether you would view the person as working with feeling, thoughts or at the concrete level.

Example one

> 'I work very hard. I often work overtime and tend to overdo it. Most of my colleagues work fairly hard, too. I suppose that we all do more than we have to. Mind you, it's important to me to work hard. That way, I make sure that we always get the things that we want for the home. We always manage to have one holiday abroad every year. There was a time when we didn't have any holidays at all. Plenty of the people we know don't have them.'

Example two

> 'I suppose I have inherited some of my personality from my mother. I often wonder how she copes. She seems so defensive. It's as though she has built a wall around herself and doesn't want to come out. I think she has probably always been like this. I suppose that she has passed some of that onto me. A process of socialization perhaps.'

Example three

> 'I find it very hard to take. I get upset very easily and don't feel I can trust myself. I always feel that I get a raw deal. I know that other people get upset easily but I just don't know why I am like this. It's as though people enjoy getting me upset. I don't like it – I know that.'

Consider yourself for a moment. Which level do you tend to work at? Do you tend to talk a lot about feelings, about your thoughts and theories or about actual events? Figure 4.1 below summarizes the different levels.

Counselling involves balancing the three elements so that what we feel links to what we think and both link to what actually happens. This model opens up various ideas about the purpose of counselling. In the end, the client must be able to make a difference to what happens to him or her at the concrete level. No amount of feeling and thinking is sufficient. In the end, what matters is that we do

The emotional level What I feel may happen What I feel about what does happen What I would like to happen How I feel about the world *Feelings*
The thinking level What I think may happen What I think about what does happen What I think should happen What I think about the world *Thoughts*
The concrete level What actually does happen The way the world is *Real life examples*

Figure 4.1 Three aspects of the counselling process

something. Sometimes, though, people are happier to stay in the domains of feelings and thoughts. Changing behaviour is often much more difficult. On the other hand, we do not just observe concrete things. We have thoughts and feelings about them too. Sometimes, what is important is what I feel about what is happening to me. Sometimes, it is vital that I can develop a theory about what is happening.

Guy Claxton (1984) summarizes some of these issues well when he suggests that we all make predictions about what will happen next: we all predict the way that the world *will* be. Claxton suggests, though, that what happens next is the way the world really is. Problems arise if our theory or feelings about the world have very little in common with the concrete facts about how the world really is. Consider the following examples which highlight both the prediction aspect of our thinking and how we feel when our predictions are not matched by the way the world is.

Example one

> 'I'm going to ask him tomorrow. I think he will say 'Yes'. If he doesn't though. I won't be too upset. I know he likes to say 'yes' when he can. If he doesn't, he must have a good reason.' (Predicting what will happen next).

Example two

> 'I'm surprised at you! I always thought you were a nice person. I didn't expect you to react in that way. It's changed the way I feel about you now. I'm sorry I asked you in the first place.' (Prediction is not matched by the way the world is.)

The three-layer model offered here owes much to the writings of the personal construct psychologist, George Kelly (1955, 1969), the works of Guy Claxton (1984) and is also directly related to my own experiences of counselling and running therapeutic groups. I have found that, as a general rule, it pays to hold each of the three levels in balance. That way, we not only notice how we think and feel but we also pay attention to what actually happens, too. Too much thinking and feeling and not enough doing can make us unrealistic and can lead to disappointment. On the other hand, as Socrates pointed out: 'the unexamined life is not worth living'.

Questions for reflection and discussion

- What are the advantages and disadvantages of the client-centred approach to counselling?
- Are nurses better at being prescriptive rather than client-centred?
- What sort of counsellor are you?'

5

Outline of the model

The subtitle of this book is *a guide to practice in nursing*. This chapter outlines a model (Figure 5.1) and offers an overview of it. The point of the model is to suggest how the counselling relationship may be structured. What are its pros and cons? These are listed below.

Pros

- It offers clear structure
- It identifies stages in the counselling relationship
- It is not biased towards a particular theory of counselling (i.e. client-centred, analytical or any other sort)

Stage One: Meeting the client
Stage Two: Agreeing a contract
Stage Three: Exploring the issues
Stage Four: Identifying priorities
Stage Five: Helping with feelings
Stage Six: Exploring alternatives
Stage Seven: Ending the relationship

Figure 5.1 Model for the structure of a counselling relationship

- It can be useful as a training guide
- It can serve as a check list of ways of counselling.

Cons

- It could be taken too literally. There is a danger in presenting a model like this that people may think that 'this is the way you do counselling'. In practice, counselling is always varied and often unpredictable. This is just *one* model: it is not *the* model.
- It might be seen as an oversimplification of the counselling process. On the other hand, you have to start somewhere. As noted in the previous objection, counselling is varied and different each time it happens. Anyone who has not done any counselling needs a framework from which to develop skills. The model offers such a framework.

The model

The model offers seven stages. Why seven and not 18 or three? First, seven stages are reasonably easy to remember. No model that cannot be remembered is likely to be used in practice. No one is likely to remember 18 stages. Equally, a three-stage model will not allow for the breakdown of the whole process into reasonably manageable parts. It is hoped then, that a seven-stage model allows for the complexity of counselling while maintaining an easy to remember format.

The model starts with the fact of meeting the client and ends with the dissolution of the relationship. In between, a clear set of stages is discussed. Again, in real life, sometimes the stages overlap. This need not be a problem, the model is there to serve as a heuristic device, a learning aid and an outline of how to proceed.

In this introduction to the model, I have presented each stage in terms of:

- Issues: what is involved in this stage?
- Problems: what difficulties might be encountered in this stage?
- Skills: what, specifically, do I need to learn in this stage?

In the chapters that come after this one, each stage is explored in much greater detail. It will be useful, at times, to return to this chapter to brush up on where each stage fits into the overall model.

Stage one: meeting the client

Every relationship starts with the meeting of two people. This stage identifies the process of beginning the counselling relationship.

Issues

- How are introductions best handled?
- What do you say in the early stages of counselling?
- What happens if I am nervous?
- Will I be able to help?

Problems

- What if I don't like the person in front of me?
- How do I cope with my own anxiety?
- What happens if I don't know what to say?

Skills

- Introductions
- Listening
- Attending.

Stage two: agreeing a contract

The counselling relationship is different to ordinary relationships. It is more than conversation and yet not quite friendship. The use of a contractual arrangement can help to structure the process of helping another person.

Issues

- What is expected of me?
- How should I structure the relationship?

Problems

- What if I am overwhelmed?
- What if I don't think I can help?

Skills

- Planning
- Structuring
- Listening.

Stage three: exploring the issues

Before anything else happens, it is necessary to hear the client's story. Without exploring the larger picture it is difficult to know how to begin to help the other person.

Issues

- What is really involved in listening to another person?
- How do I get someone to talk about themselves?

Problems

- What if I get stuck?
- What if my attention wanders?

Skills

- Listening
- Attending
- Drawing out.

Stage four: identifying priorities

We cannot take on the whole of another person's life. It is necessary in counselling, as in most things, to seek out priorities.

Issues

- Whose priorities?
- Which ones should I choose?

Problems

- How do you get someone to identify priorities?

Skills

- Brainstorming
- Listening
- Attending.

Stage five: helping with feelings

Counselling can sometimes be about exploring emotions. This stage identifies some of the difficulties and some of the skills surrounding the question of personal feelings.

Issues

- What is the nature of feelings?
- Why help with them at all?

Problems

- How do I help someone with their feelings?
- What happens when feelings are bottled up?

Skills

- Emotional release
- Listening
- Attending.

Stage six: exploring alternatives

Once priorities have been identified and feelings explored, it is time for the client to make decisions about what to do next. This stage is about deciding on what needs to be done. It is a critical stage for after it the client has to *change* if his or her life situation is also to change.

Issues

- What is the 'bottom line' in counselling?
- What really needs to happen next?

Problems

- How will I identify the real alternatives?

Skills

- Clarifying
- Focusing
- Listening
- Attending.

Stage seven: ending the relationship

Counselling relationships have a life. That life ends at a certain point. This stage explores the questions surrounding the ending of the counselling relationship.

Issues

- What if I am really involved with the other person?
- Why say goodbye?

Problems

- What if I am too involved?
- What if the client is too attached?

Skills

- Closure
- Saying goodbye
- Listening
- Attending.

What is common to each stage is the need to develop effective and excellent listening and attending skills. The heart of the counselling relationship is listening. If you can listen and not judge, if you can listen and refrain from talking back and if you can listen and not feel compelled to rush in to fix things, then you are already on the way to becoming a very effective counsellor.

Learning the model

Counselling was never learned out of a book. It is learned through doing, but through doing that is informed. This book can offer some information to get you started and to help you to reflect on aspects of the counselling process. It can also lead you to other references and other sources. What the model can do is to offer you structure for thinking about your counselling practice and your need for more theory. I feel that two principles are essential in counselling: simplicity and structure. On the one hand, it is important not to get too bogged down with complicated theories about how people's minds work or what they might really mean when they say things. In the end, what is important is that we listen and we listen some more. No amount of theory will necessarily change a person's circumstances. This is where the simplicity comes in.

Structure, on the other hand, can readily complement that simplicity. Paradoxically, structure can allow us freedom. Once we know *what* we are doing, *why* we are doing it and what we can expect the *outcome* to be, we are more likely to feel confident to experiment and to relax. A certain amount of structure can also help when we are stuck. The structure of this model can mean that we have certain signposts throughout the process of counselling. They may not always be completely accurate but they do give us some idea about where we are in a relationship and what we should do next.

Using the model in practice

The model described and discussed in this book has a variety of applications and these can be listed as follows:

- It can be used to identify the particular stages of the counselling process
- It can be used to clarify the skills that are needed at any particular stage of the counselling process
- It can be used to help you to assess and to evaluate your own skills, in terms of both strengths and deficits
- It can be used as a training guide. Teachers and trainers can use it to structure training courses and workshops.

It is worth saying again that it is *a* model and not *the* model. There are numerous ways of counselling and of thinking about counselling. The one described here is fairly straightforward and not unnecessarily complicated. Nor does it offer allegiance to one particular psychological theory.

Developing your own style

In the end, you will abandon the model. This is as it should be. We all have our own style. No one does things according to the book. Practice and experience show you other ways of doing things and other ways of helping people. The point of the model is to identify *some* ways of helping. I recommend that you use it as a learning tool and as a baseline for occasionally checking your counselling. I find it useful to reflect, every so often, on what I am doing when I am counselling. What I hope to find is that I am following the model *in principle* but not necessarily to the letter. In other words, I hope to find that I have not slipped back merely to talking and offering advice but that I observe the principles outlined in each stage of the model. Sometimes the *ordering* of the stages changes. Sometimes, a particular stage is missed out. It is hoped though, the model has a range of convenience that makes it applicable in a wide range of counselling situations. Use it, discard it and then go back to it. This, in the end, is what experiential learning, or learning from life experience, is all about.

Questions for reflection and discussion

- What are the advantages and disadvantages of the model?
- Could you use the model in practice?
- Is a model of counselling taught in the college of school in which you trained?

6

Stage one: meeting the client

Stage One: Meeting the client
Stage Two: Agreeing a contract
Stage Three: Exploring the issues
Stage Four: Identifying priorities
Stage Five: Helping with feelings
Stage Six: Exploring alternatives
Stage Seven: Ending the relationship

Initial impressions

Whether we like it or not, we are all affected by the immediate impression we have of someone when we first meet them. That impression would seem to be based on objective fact: they are there, they are dressed in a certain way; they have a particular accent; they use particular facial expressions, their hair is a certain length and so on. Closer reflection, of course, reveals that no such objectivity exists: we are basing the way we *see* those aspects of the person on what *we* think about them. Our own beliefs about the appropriate way to dress, how a person should talk and so forth are all based on our past experience, our value systems and our personal beliefs. Consider, for example, the two following first meetings.

1 You are working on a hospital ward. David James, an 18-year-old boy comes into the ward for admission for minor surgery. This is a description of him.

David is tall and thin. He is wearing a leather jacket that is covered in badges and hand-drawn pictures and slogans. Underneath the jacket, he is wearing a tee shirt with the name of a heavy metal band on it. He is also wearing faded jeans and lace up boots. He has shoulder length hair and is chewing gum.
Question: what is David like?

2 You are at a rock concert with a friend, Andrew. This is a description of him.

Andrew is about the same age as you and dressed casually. He has longish hair and is wearing a white tee shirt and jeans. The tee shirt has the name of a band on it.
Question: what is Andrew like?

It would seem that our impressions of people are based not only on our personal beliefs and previous experience but also on our expectations and on the context in which people occur. In the above examples, we may expect our friends to wear certain sorts of clothes to a rock concert. We may not expect people to wear similar sorts of clothes when coming into hospital. The problem with these sorts of *attributions* is that we do more than simply notice what people are wearing, we also begin to make *judgements* about them. We assume that they are a certain type of person. We may even judge them in terms of good or bad. Notice, if you will, how common this is. Most of us do it every day. As we watch people around us we find it convenient to slot them into certain categories: intelligent, good looking, shifty, lazy and so on. Labels of this sort are never just *descriptions* (and they are, anyway, rarely accurate descriptions), they are also *evaluations* of other people. Think, now, of these situations and what assumptions and judgements you might make of the people concerned:

- A teacher or lecturer who wears jeans to work in a school or college where suits and collars and ties are the norm.
- A nurse who personalizes his or her uniform in some way in order to make it more his or her own.
- A group leader or facilitator of a weekend workshop on counselling skills who wears a suit.

The point, as we shall see, is to find out *from the person* who they are. Such an account is, arguably, much more important in counselling than any set of prejudices, beliefs or theories that we may bring to bear.

Checking for personal identification

When we meet someone for the first time, something odd sometimes happens. They remind us of someone else. We have probably all had that experience. What is more odd, though, is that when we meet people, they nearly always remind us of someone. The problem is that we sometimes do not notice this happening. The skill, here, is to run this simple check each time we meet a person that we are going to counsel. Ask these questions:

- Of whom does this person remind me?
- In what ways is he or she similar to that other person?
- In what ways is he or she different to that person?

This identity checking is important. Without it, we can fall into an almost unconscious trap of imagining that the person we are with really is the person they remind us of. An example of this is when someone does something out of character. We say to them 'You surprise me. I never thought that you would say something like that'. Perhaps what we are really saying is something like, 'You remind me of someone else. They would not have talked like that'.

Checking stereotypes

Linked to this resemblance problem, is the one of assuming things about other people because of the way they look, dress or talk. We all make assumptions of this sort all of the time. Much of the time, this is a reasonable thing to do. For instance, it is important that we can assume that a person who dressed like a policeman *is* a member of the force.

On the other hand, it is easy to attribute things to people far beyond the evidence that we have. For example, we may assume that someone who wears a leather jacket and torn jeans is likely to hold certain sorts of values. We may even assume that they drink or take drugs. Nor do we restrict ourselves to such obvious stereotypes. Often, we make assumptions about people based on almost no data. Consider, for example, how often you have played the game of 'guessing what the person in front of you does for a living'. We are quite good at slotting people into pigeon holes.

As with the skill of separating the person in front of us from a person we have known (described in the previous section), so, too, must be learn to disassociate our attributions from the real person who is in front of us. People sometimes conform to stereotypes but often they do not. Question: to what degree do you fit a stereotype? Second question: do you mind people making assumptions about you?

Sometimes, nurse training and education can be a problem. Most nurses are trained to observe people and to draw tentative conclusions from what they observe. They are encouraged to notice signs and symptoms. With personal problems and emotional issues the situation is different. It is not possible to read people for their problems. George Kelly offered a useful piece of advice on this issue. He said that, 'If you want to know what someone is about, ask them, they might just tell you' (Kelly, 1969). The point is not to observe people and draw conclusions. The point is to *ask* people about themselves. Their account of their problems is likely to be much more important than any assumptions that you may make about them.

Initial anxiety

It has been suggested that anxiety is *always* present when two people meet to talk (Sullivan, 1955). This seems to be true even when the two people are friends or if the conversation is likely to be a pleasant one. Consider, for example, anticipating the following conversations. Try to imagine that you are going to have one of these types of conversations in about 10 minutes time. Try to notice how you would be feeling.

- Meeting a new boy or girl friend
- Meeting a friend that you have not seen for a few months
- Meeting a person you work with but at the local pub
- Meeting your boss at his or her house
- Meeting a psychiatrist at an outpatients appointment.

Reflect, particularly, on the last situation. Why might such a meeting be anxiety making? The clues are not difficult to identify. We associate psychiatrists with mental ill health; we assume that they 'know something about the mind'; we are wary about being thought of as mad; we are concerned that we might be diagnosed; we want to create a certain impression, and so on.

Think, now, about your own reputation. You are a nurse. You are thought to know something about illness. You may know something about people's problems. Also, anyone talking to you in a counselling capacity is going to be revealing themselves to you. What will you do with the information that is offered? All of these issues cause anxiety in the person who is coming to you for counselling.

Added to all this is your own anxiety. A whole range of issues crop up here. What will the client think of you? What will you say? What if you dry up? What if things go wrong? and so on.

Beneath these professional anxieties is a whole range of personal ones, too. When we meet another person, we become aware that we are offering ourselves to them. Just as we are evaluating them on various levels and as people, so, too, are they evaluating us. The whole process of meeting another person face to face can be an anxiety provoking one.

Opening the conversation

How do you start a conversation? This is such a fundamental question that it is not usually asked. Not many nurse teachers teach nurses how to start talking to another person. It is taken for granted that you know how to. Anyone, though, who has undertaken mental health training or placement will know how difficult it is to walk up to someone and start a conversation. Often in nursing, the fact that you are doing something makes the conversation easier to start. In counselling, you will often be faced just with the person on his or her own. You will be required to begin. How do you do it?

No surprises here. I am not going to offer you a formula for starting a conversation, either. What you say and how you say it will depend on many factors, including:

- Current fashion in greeting
- Regional variations
- Your age
- Your personal preference
- Your status with regard to the other person.

What I do suggest, though, is that you reflect on what you could say and what you might not say. It is worth considering, quite carefully, a range of possible 'openers' that you could use. If you practise these a little, you will no longer be stuck for something to say. I can tell you what I say, but I guarantee that it is unlikely to suit you. On meeting a person whom I am likely to counsel, for the first time, I tend to say: 'Hello, I'm Philip Burnard. You must be (name). It's good to meet you. Sit down and let's talk through a few things.'

This format ensures that the person knows who I am. It lets him know that I know his name. It also helps him to decide on how he is going to refer to me. By offering my full name, I give them the choice of addressing me by my first name or in a more formal way. As we progress, though, I would always encourage the other person to call me by my first name. The opening statement is affirmative and also indicates action. I find that this sort of statement (and I do not always use exactly these words) is useful for making sure that we both know who we are, where we are and what we are going to do next.

Think carefully about your opening statement. It is your opportunity to put the other person at his or her ease. It is also the client's introduction to you as a person. She is likely to be nervous. You are likely to be anxious. In suggesting action ('let's talk about a few things') you offer both a means of starting and sound as though you know where the conversation is going next.

The 'talking about a few things', in my case, is always a question of deciding about time, length of meetings and so on. These sorts of issues are discussed in greater detail in the next chapter. The point, here, is that the conversation does not suddenly become a counselling one. There are other things to do before settling down to a counselling relationship. At this stage, it is not even clear if counselling will or will not take place. All this is, is an initial introduction and a first meeting of two people who may or may not continue to meet each other.

Can you help?

As you get to know the other person, the key question is simply this: can you help them? This is not so easy as it first appears. The newcomer to counselling is often prone to feel that, armed with a range of counselling skills, they can help anyone. Sometimes, this is not the case. A short list of people that *I* would be doubtful about helping through counselling include the following:

- A person who actively talks of suicide
- A person who is suffering from an eating disorder of such severity that it is an immediate danger to their physical health
- A person about whom I am concerned may be suffering from a mental illness of the psychotic sort – schizophrenia or manic depressive psychosis
- A person who is plagued by obsessive thoughts which he or she cannot easily control or manage
- A person who is currently misusing drugs or dependent on alcohol.

This is a personal and short list. I am not suggesting that people who fall into one or more of these categories might not be helped by counselling. I am suggesting that *I* would not immediately think of offering myself as counsellor: other help may be of far more use to them. It is important, then, to know when to refer people on. It is less than helpful to raise people's hopes if you are unlikely to be able to help them. Equally, it is important to know *how* to refer people to other helping agencies. So, in order to make this easier, consider the following questions and find out the necessary information for yourself, if you do not have it already:

- How would you ensure that someone was able to seek psychiatric help if he wanted it?
- What are the procedures for referring someone to a social worker for more help or advice?
- Who is the occupation health adviser in your organization and how would you refer someone to them?

A person who works as a counsellor needs to know his or her limitations. He or she also needs to know what sorts of people he or she *can* help. Here is a personal list of *some* personal issues that I would be prepared to talk through with another person. Again, it is *my* list. I am not suggesting that it would necessarily suit you but it might be helpful to consider your own list and even to write it down:

- A person who has been bereaved and wants to talk through his or her feelings
- A person who has mixed feelings about his or her spiritual beliefs and feels the need to clarify them
- A person who is having problems with his or her personal relationships
- A person who is worried about his or her sexuality

- A person who feels that he or she 'bottles up' emotions and wants to explore them
- A person who is anxious or mildly depressed
- A person who is experiencing a loss of meaning in life
- A person who is concerned about his or her career
- A person who is worried about his or her course work
- A person who wonders whether or not psycotherapy might be the answer to some personal problems.

The last issue is an important one. Sometimes, counselling can be the means to deciding whether or not it really is *counselling* that a person wants or more detailed *psychotherapy*. Again, it is important that the counsellor is able to let go, know his or her limitations and be prepared to help a person make the decision to seek psychotherapy if this seems appropriate.

Noticing the levels

Three levels of counselling are discussed in this book: the feeling level, the thinking level and the concrete level. Notice how some people tend to say 'I feel . . .' while others say 'I think . . .'. Still others tend to avoid talking about their thoughts and feelings but talk, instead about things that actually happen. As part of the process of meeting a person, it is interesting to note the degree to which they talk about feelings, thoughts and theories, or actual events. A person who talks mostly at one level, may be ignoring the others. This may or may not be a form of defence. Consider these examples:

> 'I feel very mixed up. Sometimes, I wonder what is happening. I get this odd feeling that something is happening. I'm not always sure what it is but it makes me feel very uncomfortable.'

The problem, here, is exactly what is the problem. Nothing specific has been talked about.

> 'I think I may be the sort of person who rationalizes everything. I think I need to put things into categories. I expect I feel safer when I do this. It helps me to sort everything out. The problem is, it may be a little too neat.'

The problem, here, is how does this person feel about himself. All we have at the moment is a theory.

> 'When I get to work, I work very hard. I usually keep going all the time. I rarely stop for lunch. When I do, it's a short break. Mind you, I don't normally eat very much anyway.'

The problem, here, is what does this person feel about what is happening? What do they think about? All we have at the moment is a description of what happens.

The examples above indicate the three levels of orientation to the world: The first person seems to work mostly at a feelings level; the second person tends to work at a thinking level; the third tends to work at a concrete level. Noting this at an early stage in the relationship is quite useful as a guide to what can be done in the counselling sessions.

Reflect on yourself for a moment. What sort of person are you? Do you work on a feeling, thinking or concrete level? My guess is that you will be tempted to say, straight away, 'I work on all three: what a stupid question!' Reflect a little more. I suggest that you may well find that one of the three predominates.

What not to do in this stage

- Don't rush
- Don't get too deep too quickly
- Don't take on counselling if you know you are out of your depth.

When not to start counselling

- When the other person expresses suicidal thoughts
- When the other person is clearly very disturbed
- When the other person asks to see someone else
- When you feel unable to help
- When you feel it right to refer on.

When to refer on directly

- When the other person expresses suicidal thoughts
- When the other person threatens harm to another person
- When the person is clearly in danger.

Activities for learning this stage

Activity one: in the next few days, notice people meeting each other. Pay particular attention to the *behaviour* they demonstrate.

Activity two: experiment with your own introductions. In the next few weeks, try introducing yourself to other people using a range of approaches. Try the direct, eye-to-eye approach as well as the more reticent approach. Notice which sort of introduction you feel most comfortable with and notice how other people respond to you in the various situations.

Questions for reflection and discussion

- What are the most difficult parts of meeting people for you?
- What behaviours do you associate with people who are good at introductions?
- Are nurses generally good at introducing themselves?

7

Stage two: agreeing the contract

Stage One: Meeting the client
Stage Two: Agreeing a contract
Stage Three: Exploring the issues
Stage Four: Identifying priorities
Stage Five: Helping with feelings
Stage Six: Exploring alternatives
Stage Seven: Ending the relationship

Having agreed that you *can* help the person you are with, through counselling, the next thing to do is to set a contract. The word can mean different things in different contexts. In this case it refers to the idea that both you and the client should be clear about the nature of your relationship. Deciding upon the contract in the relationship can ensure that you have a structure within which to work and that you are both clear about what the relationship *does* and *does not* offer. The elements of that contract are:

- Time
- Place
- Confidentiality
- Length of the counselling relationship
- What is expected
- What is offered.

There are, of course, other elements that you may wish to think about in considering a contract. Essentially, though, you need to be clear about for how long you will meet, where you will meet, how long you anticipate the counselling relationship to last, whether or not it will be a confidential one and what is expected and offered in the relationship.

The contract is not a written one: it is a verbal agreement and clarification takes place between the two people involved. Also, it cannot contain aims or objectives. Before counselling has occurred, it is impossible to set particular goals. One of the purposes of counselling is to explore the client's world and to try to identify the sorts of things that are making life difficult. Those things cannot be known before counselling begins and aims and objectives cannot, therefore, be set.

Time

How long should a counselling session last? Traditionally, counselling meetings last about one hour although there is nothing particularly magical about this figure. One hour does, however, allow the client to open up and talk fairly freely. Also, it is not so long as to exhaust both the client and the counsellor. What is important is to establish, from the start, how long each session will last. Why?

First, as nurses, we all lead fairly busy lives. Very few people can offer an open-ended amount of time to another person. Also, how could you judge when to stop? If you have a pre-set contract to meet for a certain amount of time, once or twice a week, then you are both clear on when the counselling will start and when it will stop.

Second, people tend to disclose what is *really* important to them, towards the end of a counselling session. Often, this takes place at an almost unconscious level. It seems unlikely that anyone sets out to disclose only towards the end. The fact is, though, that this is what happens. If the client knows when the counselling session is to end, it will offer a signpost to when it is 'safe' to disclose. If the session is completely open-ended, neither the client nor the counsellor knows when the end will come. Therefore, it is often possible for the client to leave the session without having talked about the really important issues. It is as though the structuring of time in this way allows the client freedom to talk about what is really worrying them.

Once the time limit has been agreed, it is important to stick to it. It is often tempting to think on a particular day, that you have plenty of time and therefore the conversation can overrun the set time limit. It is best, whenever possible, to stick to the agreed time. If you do not, there will come a time when you cannot afford to run over (perhaps because, on that day, you have another appointment straight after the present one). On the day that you stick to the agreed time, after so many weeks of being flexible, it is likely that the client will feel that this is a result of something that he or she has said. No one likes a fairly informal relationship suddenly becoming a more formal one. If you *suddenly* find yourself having to return to the timing contract, it is likely to be seen as a return to formality. It is usually better to be consistent and to make sure that the time issue is adhered to on every occasion.

On this point, notice any tendency you have to *underrun* slightly or to *overrun* on the time issue. Sometimes, anxiety about what *might* be talked about causes the counsellor to cut the conversation down by a few minutes. Sometimes, too, anxiety about not letting the client have his or her say causes the conversation to overrun. It may sound a little inflexible, but a lot of problems can be avoided by sticking very consistently to the time agreed!

When you *are* setting the time element of the contract, make sure that you can reasonably offer the amount of time that you are agreeing. The usual hour is fine if you can find an hour a week in your schedule. It is not fine if it means that in order to do that you are having to work into your own free time. As suggested above, there is nothing magical about the hour. If you cannot reasonably offer an hour, make it half an hour. Once set, though, be consistent and stick to the time agreed.

Place

Where will you meet for counselling? Few clinical environments have spare quiet rooms for counselling (although a number are now developing this sort of facility). If you work in the community, the meeting place is often fairly obvious – the person's home. However, when possible, there is a lot to be said for meeting on neutral territory: a room away from the client's home and away from your own work area. This allows you to establish a safe place which the client comes to associate with talking. Think about this for a few moments. Would you feel happy talking about personal issues inside your own home? You might, but perhaps it is more likely that you would find it easier to talk in a place that was a little less personal. If possible, then, find a room which is going to be available to you both, each week, for the time that you have both agreed.

The other point about the neutral territory is that it is usually possible to ensure that it is somewhere where neither of you is going to be interrupted. If you counsel in the clinical setting, it is quite possible that people will interrupt you for medicine keys, to take telephone calls and so on. If you counsel in the client's home, other sorts of interruptions are likely. The neutral meeting place can help to overcome these problems.

Nor does such a meeting place have to be a formal one. You might, for example, agree to meet in a coffee area which you know to be quiet at a particular time each week. Or you may want to meet in a local park. Few of us have ready access to the ideal counselling setting with comfortable chairs in a quiet room, with no 'phone and no interruptions. In the end, we nearly all have to compromise. It is important, though, once you have agreed to meet in a certain place, to stick to that meeting place throughout your sessions. In this way, you both come to associate that place with counselling and with the process of talking about personal issues. If the environment changes from week to week, you may find that you have to keep redeveloping the relationship.

If, on the other hand, you *can* establish the ideal setting (or you are asked to advise on what would be the ideal), the following issues should be considered:

- Privacy
- Sound proofing
- Congenial surroundings
- Two chairs of equal height
- Freedom from interruption.

One other point needs consideration. That is the issue of where you both sit in terms of the nearest window. Consider this for a moment. If you sit (in normal light) in front of a window, while the client sits opposite you, it is likely that you will be sitting in shadow. This means that the client will not be able to see you clearly and that you will appear as a mysterious voice talking out of the shadow! This is hardly the environment in which to engender trust and confidence. Exactly the opposite problem occurs if the client sits in front of the window – you will not be able to see him or her clearly. If this happens, you will not be able to see all of the non-verbal aspects of communication which form such an essential part of what we say to each other. Ideally, then, try to arrange the furniture so that neither of you has his or her back to the window.

Confidentiality

Can you offer a confidential relationship to the person whom you are counselling? At first sight, the issue may seem cut and dried: it would seem that you *must* be able to. On the other hand, consider the following conversation:

> **Client**: 'Can we talk in complete confidence? I need to know that what I say to you will not go any further.'
> **Nurse**: 'Yes, of course. Whatever you say to me won't go any further. You know you can trust me.'
> **Client**: 'Thank goodness for that. I have decided that I can't stand it any more and I'm going to take an overdose tomorrow . . . I really am. I'm going to finish it, once and for all . . .'.

This is, of course, a worst-possible scenario but not an impossible one. The question arises as to how the conversation might be continued. Does the nurse, having heard the client's statement, continue to offer confidentiality, with all of the difficulties that that decision may entail? Or does she try to renegotiate the issue of confidentiality? If so, what happens if the client follows this by saying:

> 'No. It's really important to me that you don't tell anyone. I wouldn't have told you if I thought I couldn't trust you . . .'.

Both client and counsellor are in an impossible situation. How could this have been avoided? Perhaps by avoiding the 'totally confidential' counselling contract. This means that nothing that is discussed in the counselling relationship is passed on to another person unless the issue is first discussed with the client. In other words, no other person is told anything that they do not need to know, thus most of the counselling relationship does remain a confidential one. Such an intermediate contract avoids dangerous pitfalls such as the one outlined above, but it also ensures that the privacy of the client is honoured.

One other observation may be made at this point. Most people, by the time they have decided to talk through their problems with another person, will talk about them regardless of whether or not *complete* confidentiality is established. As the philosopher, John-Paul Sartre, noted: most people choose the person they want to talk to because they *know* what sort of relationship they can expect (Sartre, 1954). In other words, people decide fairly early on whether or not they can *trust* you. Also, of course, the nurse's *Code of Professional Conduct* (Burnard and Chapman, 1988) notes that you must not discuss details of client's problems with people other than those required to know. In this way, then, both client and counsellor are protected both from themselves and from each other.

Life is rarely as clear cut as this. Recently, I gave a talk to some students on this question of confidentiality and made the statement that I would not, readily, offer a completely confidential in counselling relationship. This was challenged by one of the students who said: 'If someone *really* wanted to talk to you and would only do so if you *did* offer confidentiality, what would you do?' I said that I would probably go ahead and offer them that confidentiality on the basis that they would appear to be in fairly desperate need to talk to someone. The day after the discussion with the students, the student who had raised the question came to see me and asked me for just such an assurance. I had, of course, to offer it. It transpired that nothing in the conversations that followed caused either of us alarm at having entered into that contract. In the end, it has to be acknowledged that there will always be exceptions to rules of ethics and professional practice. The *general* rule, though, remains: do not readily offer a confidential relationship if you feel that, in doing so, you may put yourself or your client at risk.

Length of the counselling relationship

For how long should you continue to meet another person for counselling? Four weeks, three months, two years? As with the timing element of the contract, it is often useful to set a time limit on the counselling relationship. This may seem a little harsh and it may be argued that it is impossible to know how long it will take to help another person with their problems. This may be true, but it is also true that most of us cannot offer indefinite support to another person.

One useful and appropriate approach to this issue is to have a *series* of time-frames. Thus, it can be agreed, at the first meeting, that you and the client will meet each week for a month. After one month, you will both review what has happened and evaluate the contract. This gives the client reasonable reassurance that he or she can meet you on a regular basis and it also sets a limit.

At the end of the first month, it is useful to reflect back over that month and decide what is to be done next. Are you to continue as you are? Are there to be changes in the *style* of the counselling? Should the counselling relationship be terminated? All of these issues can be dealt with on the fourth meeting. At that point, too, you can set another time-frame: perhaps for a longer period, perhaps for another month. Once you have established this aspect of the contract, it is important to make a note of it and to make sure that you *do* review the relationship after the agreed span of time.

What is expected?

People come to the counselling relationship with all sorts of expectations. Some come expecting advice. Some come with the notion that the counsellor will sort everything out. Yet others come believing that nothing will help and that even counselling, itself, will be a waste of time. It is important, in the early days of the relationship to explore and examine what it is that the client anticipates.

Some people may expect the counselling relationship to be one in which all sorts of medical advice is given. In certain contexts, such as family planning, genetic, or AIDS counselling, this may be appropriate but these are not the sorts of counselling that are specifically addressed in this book. If the context of the counselling is personal and emotional problems – problems of living – then it should be made clear that specific medical advice cannot be offered.

What is offered?

Just as the client has expectations, so does the counsellor. The counsellor will expect the client to talk and will want to reassure the client that he or she is allowed to talk about anything during the time that they are together. It is the client's time and, as such, that time can be used in any way the client wants. During this period, the counsellor promises to listen and not to judge. Also, though, the counsellor will need to make it clear that what is *not* offered is advice about how the client might 'put his life right'. The counsellor may also want to assure the client that the counselling relationship is not a psychotherapeutic one. It is not unusual for people to imagine that counsellors psychoanalyse people and it is necessary, sometimes, for the counsellor to reassure on this issue.

Under the heading of 'what is offered' also comes all of the issues about time and place, as discussed above. It is important that the client is under no illusions as to what the counselling relationship can offer and is clear about the structure of the process of counselling. It is also vital that the counsellor does not offer *too much*. That is to say that the counsellor retains the right to *refer on* if that appears to be necessary to both parties. Nurses working as counsellors are not psychiatrists, social workers or physicians. Any medical or other issues that cannot be worked upon during the counselling sessions must be appropriately referred to someone who *can* help. Ideally, the nurse/counsellor works in harmony and as a complement to the other medical and paramedical services and agencies.

Agreeing the contract

How is such a contract agreed? We have already noted that the contract is not (normally) a written one (although it is possible to imagine situations where both parties might prefer a written statement). If it is not a written agreement, it is important for both parties to be clear that an agreement *has* been made. The counsellor can ensure that this is the case by being very clear about the fact. The conversation, at an early stage in the relationship may go like this:

> 'Let's see what we have agreed. We will meet together once a week for an hour, for the next four weeks. After that, we will review what has happened and work out another time span. During that time, we will discuss anything that you want and I will make sure that nothing you tell me is passed on to anyone who does not need to know what we have been talking about. How does that sound to you?'
> 'Generally, that sounds OK. It will be a relief to talk to someone. I would prefer it if sometimes it was a bit less than an hour. Sometimes, I need to get away a little earlier on a Tuesday.'
> 'That's OK. Shall we agree to meet for 45 minutes, then?'
> 'Yes. That all sounds fine. Thanks.'

Changing the contract

If the original contract is clear and reasonably simple in structure, it will not, normally, need to be changed. Exceptions to this might be place and time. Sometimes, it will become necessary to change a meeting place or to adjust times. One aspect that should remain unchanged, however, is that of the question of confidentiality. It is tempting, sometimes, as the relationship deepens, to modify the relationship to a fully confidential one but this is not to be recommended, for the reasons discussed above. Once it has been agreed that the relationship will be reasonably and professionally confidential no further modification is usually necessary or advisable.

Activity for learning this stage

As you work in the ward, clinical or community setting, notice the range of contracts that exist between health care professionals and their clients. Try to observe the limits of such contracts and what happens when contracts are broken. Notice, for example, what happens when a patient exhibits behaviour that a health care professional clearly views as inappropriate. Notice, too, the sanctions that are brought to bear to reinstate the contract.

Questions for reflection and discussion

- To what degree could a contract be restrictive?
- Do you ever offer patients confidentiality?
- What are the best things about a contractual approach to counselling in nursing?

8

Stage three: exploring the issues

Stage One: Meeting the client
Stage Two: Agreeing a contract
Stage Three: Exploring the issues
Stage Four: Identifying priorities
Stage Five: Helping with feelings
Stage Six: Exploring alternatives
Stage Seven: Ending the relationship

This is the central part of the counselling relationship. The aim of this stage is to enter into the world of the client as far as possible. The idea is that the nurse listens to the client, hears his story and tries to appreciate that person's situation as *they* see it. The aim is not to identify priorities or to search for specific problems nor is it to seek solutions. All of these come later. This stage is the one of empathizing with the client and of developing as full a picture of the client's life-world as is possible.

Why not go straight for the key issues? Why not aim at identifying the problems that exist? Simply because problems do not exist in isolation. They are always related to other things. For example, the person who is concerned about the way they look does not have a problem that can simply be labelled 'problem of appearance'. Such a problem is linked to self-esteem, other members of the family, people at work, confidence in applying for jobs, getting on with other people and a whole range of other issues. It is not particularly helpful, in the early stages of counselling, to go straight for the obvious or big issues. Sometimes, the *real* problems are less obvious and less big. Also, it often happens that the things that the client initially thinks are the problems, turn out to be a cover for other, underlying problems.

I was involved in counselling someone recently who felt sure that if she could improve on her college work, she would feel happier. She worried continuously about whether or not she would ever qualify as a nurse. The presenting problem appeared to be studying. After some weeks of talking through all of this person's life issues, it became clear to both of us that what was behind the studying problem was a much deeper concern about whether or not she was acceptable to other people. The student lacked confidence, worried about whether or not she was ever going to have a boyfriend and thought that her family did not like her. It was after she was able to tell her story that these other issues emerged. Had we gone straight into discussing studying, these underlying issues may not have surfaced.

The key skills in this stage of the counselling process are non-judgemental listening and the giving of full attention. The aim, as we have noted, is to emphathize and to enter the world of the other person – to attempt to see the world as they see it. This stage is more about standing back and taking the broader view of what the client is saying than about focusing and attempting detective work.

Carl Rogers (1983) uses the phrase 'an expanding frame of reference' to describe the slow but developing understanding of the other person. It is as though we begin with almost no understanding of the person in front of us, then we get to know them a little better and the jigsaw begins to become more and more complete. It never will be complete, of course. We never can know someone completely and, anyway, they are continually changing. We can, though, get a much fuller picture than the one we started with.

The ability to suspend judgement comes into play in this stage. We are not there to criticize, moralize or judge. We are simply there to listen. This is not particularly easy. It is worth noting that we all seem to have an internal censor inside out heads when we listen to another person. As they talk, the censor tells us: 'yes, that's alright', or 'no, that's wrong' and so on. Notice how that internal censor works even as you read. My guess is that you are constantly evaluating what you are reading. That evaluation often takes the shape of whether or not what is written is right or wrong. So it is when we listen to another person. In counselling, though – and particularly in this stage – we are required to put the censor out of action and merely to take in and listen. It is rather like visiting a large house and wandering from room to room and refraining from passing judgement as to whether or not we like or dislike what we see. We are there merely to *see* the rooms.

Listening and attending

Listening is the most important skill of all. The most skilled counsellors often operate almost silently – they listen far more than they talk. I read once of a woman in an Indian town who set up a stall with a big placard in front of it which read, *I listen*. Apparently, she was never without someone in front of her stall. If we can learn really to listen to another person, we are not only on the way to becoming good counsellors but also to becoming good friends and colleagues.

Before we start a discussion of the skills of listening and attending, consider the people you know that you would call 'good listeners'. What tells you that they are good? What do they do? 'Well', you might say, 'they listen!' The point is, though, that not only do they listen, they also show that they listen. It is one thing to be a good listener, it is another to demonstrate that skill. In order that listening is effective, it must be visible.

Initially, then, it helps to adopt behaviours that show you are listening. These are not foolproof. It is quite possible to adopt the behaviours and still not listen. The point is that if we can adopt the behaviours and add the necessary relationship skills, we are completing the circle – we listen and we are seen to be listening. The behaviours are suggested by Egan (1990):

- Sit squarely. Face the client rather than sit next to him or her. Sitting facing the client means that we are able to see his or her expressions, gestures and all of the non-verbal and paralinguistic aspects of speech. Most of all, we can see their eyes and they can see ours. It may be an exaggeration (and a cliché) to say that the eyes are the windows of the soul but they do have a large part to play in communication.

- Sit in an open position. Do not fold your arms and cross your legs. On the other hand, be flexible about this. Egan was writing largely for an American audience. In the UK, it is common for most people to cross their legs when sitting down. However, the more open you can be in your posture, the more open you are likely to appear to the client.
- Lean slightly towards the other person. Do not overwhelm them but leaning towards them shows that you are with them. If you find this unlikely, try sitting with someone and leaning away from them. You will soon see the effect.
- Maintain comfortable eye contact. Do not stare and do not 'follow the client's eyes'. No one likes to feel pursued. But do be ready to take up the eye contact of the client, when he or she looks up.
- Relax. You do not have to rehearse what you want to say. You do not have to think out why the person is talking the way that they are. All you have to do is sit and listen to their story. Initially, this is often difficult. As you develop counselling skills, though, you learn to trust yourself. You begin to know that you will be able to respond once the other person has finished speaking. You will know when to respond by their eye contact. Normally, when someone in a conversation wants the other person to say something, they look at that person. Do not be too ready to rush in and fill temporary silences. Just sit and listen and relax.

Egan suggests the acronym SOLER as an easy method of remembering these behaviours:

- S : sit squarely
- O : open position
- L : lean forward
- E : eye contact
- R : relax.

Remember, though, that cultural differences come into play when listening takes place. These differences are particularly evident when it comes to eye contact. People from far eastern countries, for example, will tend not to make eye contact with people they consider to be occupying a superior role. West Indians often do not make eye contact when they are *talking* but only when they are *listening*. It is impossible in a book of this size to consider all the possible regional variations, but do not assume that the SOLER behaviours will necessarily be appropriate in all situations. They key issue, when counselling people from another culture is to take the lead from them. Notice how they respond to you and do your best to acknowledge and respect the differences. Also, if you are likely to counsel lots of people from different cultures, read as much as you can about those cultures and talk to other health care professionals who have had cross-cultural experience. The most important thing is to avoid *ethnocentricity*: the idea that the way that you do things, in your culture, is necessarily the right way.

Three zones of attention

Listening behaviours are linked to the internal state of the counsellor. The counsellor is not simply using a set of behaviours, he or she is also doing something inside the head. This is where the concept of awareness is useful. Figure 8.1 illustrates three zones of attention. In zone one, the client's attention is focused directly on the client. The counsellor whose attention is in zone one is fully alert, noticing how the client looks and fully taking in the words that the client is using.

As people talk, however, attention wanders into zone two. We think about what we are seeing and hearing. It is in this zone that the censor, described above, resides. Somehow, we have to learn to silence the censor and to return out attention to zone one. This can be a conscious effort. It is quite possible to notice what is happening to your attention and to redirect it. Try it now. Stop reading this book and allow your attention to drift into zone two: become preoccupied with your own thoughts and feelings. Notice the degree to which your censor is at work and put it out of action. Then return to the book and concentrate fully on what you read. In doing this you are consciously moving from zone one to zone two and back again.

<table>
<tr><td rowspan="2">ZONE ONE

Attention is focused on the client</td><td>ZONE TWO

Attention is focused on your own thoughts and feelings</td></tr>
<tr><td>ZONE THREE

Attention is focused on fantasy and on what you BELIEVE is the case</td></tr>
</table>

Figure 8.1 The three zones of attention

Zone three is more problematic. It is here that we 'make things up'. It is the zone of fantasy. When our thoughts and feelings are not satisfied by what we see or hear, we simply fill in the details and fantasize. Again, this can be demonstrated fairly easily. Stop reading this book and move into zone two. Note what you are thinking and feeling. Now, do something else: think about the writer of this book. What do I look like? Unless you have met me, you have just moved into the zone of fantasy! You have no means of knowing how I look and yet you are able to offer some sort of answer to the question.

We often work in the domain of fantasy. When someone walks in the room we do not simply note what they look like, we go beyond that. We make a quick (and fallacious) assessment of them. We note whether or not we are likely to like them. We establish whether or not they are like us. We may put them into all sorts of other categories. And yet all of this categorization is built on almost no factual input!

The point of all this for the counsellor is simply this: as far as possible, when sitting with the client, stay out of the zone of fantasy. Stick to what the client is telling you. Listen to what they say. If something is not clear, ask for clarification. If you suspect something to be the case, ask the client. Do not jump to conclusions and try, as far as possible, to stay in zone one; stay with the client for as long as possible. For it is in zone one that you will really get to know the patient. All you will do in zone three is invent.

Listening to the client involves two elements: external behaviours – showing that you are listening – and internal behaviours – purposely focusing your attention on the client. This combination is useful throughout the counselling relationship. If it can be sustained, it can lead to counselling becoming much more focused on the client's world than on the counsellor's belief system. In the end, what matters is what the client thinks, feels and does. The relationship, if you like, belongs to the client. The time spent counselling is time for the client to work through his or her own problems. It is not time for the counsellor to rehearse his or her own theories about human nature or about what is wrong with the client.

Using open questions

Asking questions is a major part of the task of being a counsellor. There is a world of difference, though, between the questioning of an interrogator and the questioning of a counsellor. The interrogator or even the interviewer is there to get information. The counsellor uses questions in a different sort of way. The counsellor uses questions in order to help the client and the counsellor to illuminate the client's world. It is as though the counsellor is testing the ground by saying, 'is it like this?' . . . 'or like this?' . . . The counsellor does not so much seek out information for its own sake, but more, in order to clarify. Skilful questioning is never obtrusive and certainly not intrusive. Consider the following examples and try to decide whether they might be part of a counselling process.

Example one:

'What did you do once you left home?'
'I spent some time moving from place to place. It was difficult, really, I found it difficult to settle.'
'Where did you finally settle down?'
'In the north of England. I found a small village where people seemed to accept me and I got a job and things.'
'What did you do, during that period?'
'I worked in a factory at first.'
'Were you good at work?'
'Yes, I think so. I enjoyed it, too. I always thought that I would stay in factory work.'
'But you didn't?'

Example two:

'When was your first admission to hospital?'
'It must have been in April last year.'
'What was the reason for your admission then? Can you remember?'
'I think I was told that I was having some sort of investigation . . . I can't really remember . . .'
'Was it *this* hospital?'

Example three:

'What happened once you left home?'
'I didn't settle very easily. I moved from place to place.'
'What was that period like for you?'
'It was a very difficult period. I didn't like it very much . . . at least, I always say to myself that I didn't like it. I suppose, looking back as we're talking, it can't have been all that bad . . . I mean, I survived it, didn't I?'
'But some parts of it were uncomfortable for you?'
'Yes. Some parts of it were awful. I found it difficult to know where to live. I didn't know what I wanted to do and I didn't know what I *could*

do. The whole time I was unsettled. I hardly knew anyone, so I had no friends.'
'Was that difficult?'
'Well, it was in a way. I mean, I've always been a fairly solitary person but everyone needs someone to talk to and, anyway, it meant I had few contacts on the job front. It wasn't easy at that time . . .'

It should be clear that the last example is the counselling example. What is also noticeable in that example is that the *client* talks more than the counsellor. Questioning in counselling is not only about how to ask questions, it is also about knowing when to stay silent, when to let the client think a little more before he or she carries on with a particular train of thought. As we have noted, the questioning process in counselling is more to clarify than to gather information.

Open and closed questions

It is usual to discriminate between two extremes in questioning: open and closed questions. The open question is the question which to which the counsellor cannot guess the answer. Open questions are not usually answered with one word but by a series of sentences. Thus, the following are examples of open questions:

- How do you feel about that?
- What happened after that?
- What are your thoughts about it?

Open questions are particularly useful in helping the client to open up and to expand on what he or she is saying. They are useful memory joggers and are frequently used in any stage of the counselling process, but are of particular value in exploring the client's problems and issues.

Closed questions, on the other hand, usually have a definite answer and one that the counsellor can usually make a guess at. If this is not the case, the counsellor will usually have some idea of what *sort* of answer is likely to be forthcoming. Thus, these are examples of closed questions:

- How many children do you have?
- Did you ever meet your father?
- What is your grandmother's name?

While closed questions are useful for gathering very particular pieces of information and are thus helpful in filling in the jigsaw, they can also often appear to be intrusive or just nosy. It is probably better to restrict the number of closed questions that you use. In a way, the process is self-limiting. If you *do* use too many closed questions, the conversation will tend to slow down or stop, anyway. Consider the following example:

'When did you come into hospital for the first time?'
'Earlier this year, I think . . .'
'What, in January or February?'
'February, I think it was.'
'Was it this hospital?'
'Yes.'
'Did you have an operation?'
'Yes.'
'What sort?'
'I think it was called a laparotomy.'

Too many closed questions soon lead to silence. Having made this distinction between open and closed questions, it is important to note that there are *degrees* of openness and closure in questioning. Sometimes, what appears to be an open question, becomes a closed one. Consider this example:

'How did you feel about leaving your family?'
'OK. No problem.'

Here, what seemed to the counsellor to be a open question was turned into a closed one by the client. It is worth considering why this happens. Quite often it happens because the counsellor has chosen the wrong *sort* of question to ask: that is, the wrong sort of question about the wrong sort of issue. In the example, above, it seems likely that the counsellor thought that the issue of 'leaving your family' was an important one. It also seems that the issue was not a particularly burning one for the client. The counsellor had misjudged the sort of question to ask. If you find a lot of your open questions being turned into closed ones, ask yourself whether or not you are asking the *right* questions.

Earlier, we discussed the three possible levels of exploration: the feeling level, the thinking level and the concrete level. This series of levels comes into its own under the heading of questioning. The skilful

Feeling questions How do you feel about that? What does that feel like?
Thinking questions What are you thinking? What are your thoughts about that?
Concrete questions Can you give me an example? What actually happened?

Figure 8.2 Questions for various levels

counsellor can choose to switch levels by asking questions that are aimed at the various levels (Figure 8.2). In aiming at the different levels, the questions must be very specific. Thus a thinking question needs to contain the phrase 'what do you think . . . ?' and a feeling one, 'what do you feel . . .'. Also, the counsellor needs to listen carefully to the answer, for the client can resist the changing of levels. Consider the following exchange.

'What did you feel about your job?'
'I think it was alright. It paid well and I managed to get through the work.'
'And what did you *feel* about it?'
'Feel about it? I hated it!'

In this example, the counsellor gently persisted on the 'feeling' level and the client then expressed his feelings quite forcibly. Such level switching takes patience and attention and also considerable practice. Try to notice the sorts of questions that you tend to ask of other people. Which level do you tend to work on most?

It is quite possible to combine the three levels of questioning in any particular counselling session. Sometimes it is very useful to be able to move freely between the three. An example of where a nurse is working in this way is as follows:

'what did you feel about leaving hospital?'
'I felt very vulnerable at first. I felt as though I had been thrown out . . . it was very uncomfortable for a while . . .'

'So what did you do?'
'I tried to discuss it with my husband. He tried to understand, I think, but I'm not sure that he really did. He just thought that I would be happy to be back home, which, in a way, I was. It still felt awful, though . . .'
'What sort of feelings did you have . . . ?'
'Anger. Disappointment. I felt all sorts of things. It was very confusing, really.'
'What did you think was going on?'
'I think I was trying to sort out in my own mind how I felt about the baby and how I felt about my husband. I was surprised, I think, by how *mixed* my feelings were. I had thought, before I went into hospital, that I really wanted the baby and that I was really fond of my husband. When I came back from the hospital, I found myself questioning a lot of those things. It was odd . . .'
'And upsetting?'
'Yes. Definitely.'

Questions to avoid

There are certain sorts of questions that are best not asked at all. These can be identified fairly easily in theory, but are sometimes difficult to avoid in practice. In order to avoid them it is necessary to remain clear about the *aims* of asking questions and clear about avoiding judgement. Here are some of the sorts of questions to avoid.

Loaded questions

These are questions that reveal the counsellor's own particular beliefs or prejudices about the client. An example of a loaded question is:

'Did you feel guilty about the way you treated your wife?'

The implication is that the client *should* have felt guilty. Also, however the client answers, he puts himself in a difficult position. If he says 'yes', he acknowledges guilt. If he says 'no', it sounds as though he did not feel the guilt that was appropriate! This sort of question is sometimes called a *leading* question. Perhaps the most famous leading question (which, again, would cause real difficulties, however it was answered) is:

'Have you stopped beating your wife?'

Multiple questions

Sometimes, in the quest to get things right, it is possible to roll a number of questions into one:

> 'How did you feel about being in hospital? Did you think that you were treated fairly well? Did you feel you could have managed better on your own . . . ?'

The obvious problem, here, is which question is the client supposed to answer? Try to ask only one question at a time.

Unclear questions

This is a variant of the multiple question. When we are anxious or trying hard to be clear, it is possible to do exactly the opposite and to become very muddled. Then, sometimes, our questions become very unclear:

> 'What did you do . . . I mean, what did you want to happen, sort of, before everything was sorted out at home and everything . . . ?'

As a general rule, short questions are usually more effective than lengthy ones. If you find yourself getting into a mess, *acknowledge* that you have done so and start again. Remember, it is OK to make a mess of things sometimes: it lets the client know that you are human, too.

Intrusive questions

The aim of counselling is to help the client to solve problems. The aim is not to collect all sorts of very personal data about the other person. It is sometimes tempting to want to probe the other person's life a little. Sometimes, our nosiness gets the better of us. It is important that we do not ask questions that could embarrass or offend the client, such as:

> 'Do you still feel sexually attracted to him?'

The issue of intrusiveness has to be put in context. Clearly, there are times, as the relationship develops, when such a question *might* be appropriate. However, in this early stage of the counselling process, it seems unlikely that it would be. If you feel tempted to ask very personal questions, ask *yourself* why you are asking it and what your motivation might be for asking it.

Empathy building

Empathy is the ability to enter into the other person's frame of reference: to feel as they feel. Empathy building is the process of *conveying* that shared experience with the client. Thus empathy-building statements are always tentative and also try to ensure that the counsellor is matching what the client is feeling. This is never easy but it gets easier as the relationship deepens. Sometimes, the counselling relationship is a bit like a trance that you both slowly go into and both slowly emerge from at the end of your time together. It becomes as though only the two of you exist for the time that you are talking. Any interruption, such as a phone ringing or someone else coming into the room seems an intrusion.

Empathy-building statements, then, are those that illustrate that you are matching the feelings and experience of the other person. Examples of empathy building statements are:

> 'It feels as though . . .'
> 'I get the impression that . . .'
> 'Is it the case that . . . ?'

You always know if your empathy building is not going the way you would like it. The client lets you know fairly quickly. Here is an example of a situation in which empathy-building statements are wide of the mark.

> 'It sounds as though you were quite upset during that period of your life . . .'
> 'No! On the contrary, I was very relieved to be on my own again. I was happier then than I had been for a long time.'

When this happens, it is probably best to stop attempting empathy-building statements and to concentrate on listening with greater accuracy. Sometimes, empathy-building statements do not work because the counsellor is trying too hard. When this happens, again, it is best to relax a little and allow the client to talk more. Remember: the relationship belongs to the client. The time you are together is the client's time. There is absolutely no need to rush the process and, anyway, most human relationships refuse to be rushed. You cannot force empathy: it has to be really there.

Reflection

Reflection (sometimes called echoing) is a familiar and well-known counselling strategy. Two sorts can be described. First, there is straightforward reflection of the last thing that the client said. Thus, when the client begins to falter in what he or she is saying, the counsellor repeats back the last few words that were spoken:

> 'We were happy when we lived in London. Most of our friends were there and the kids were happy. We all liked it, because we knew what was happening . . .'
> 'You knew what was happening . . .'
> 'Well, we *understood* the situation. We were all settled. Then, my wife had to move because of her job and we all found ourselves in a strange town and we didn't know a soul.'

This type of reflection acts as a simple prompt. The client is momentarily lost in the conversation and the counsellor gently nudges him back on track. It is important to note that a reflected comment should not become a *question*. It is important that the comment is reflected back with much the same tone and volume that it was uttered by the client. If it *does* become a question, it will be *answered* as a question:

> 'We all liked it, I think, because we knew what was happening . . .'
> 'You knew what was happening?'
> 'Yes'(!).

The second type of reflection is where something is reflected back from the *middle* of what the client has been saying: something that was emphasized or which appears to be an emotional issue. An example of this sort of reflection is as follows:

> 'We had been happy in London. Now we were somewhere else. My children really, really hated it. I thought they would settle down but they didn't really. I suppose none of us settled down very quickly.'
> 'Your children really hated it . . .'
> 'It was as though they were different people. In London they had been so happy and now they were being dragged away from their school and their friends and everything . . .'

Even people who have fairly monotonous voices emphasize certain things as they talk. In order to use this second, selective, form of reflection, it is important to remain very attentive and for that attention to remain 'free floating'. It is no good hanging onto a phrase in order to feed it back as a selective reflection! It is impossible to know, in advance, when the other person is likely to stop talking. Five minutes later, the selective reflection that you had planned may be 'out of date'. Thus, the need to maintain free floating attention: attention that takes everything in but which also gently shifts as the client shifts the focus of the conversation.

Reflection can be a useful way of gently encouraging the other person to continue his or her train of thought. It has to be used wisely, though. It can easily be misused and when it is, the conversation takes on a slightly odd character. It is likely, too, that the client will notice the oddness and comment on it, thus:

> 'We were happier when we moved to Liverpool. It was bigger and we were used to life in the town, anyway . . .'
> 'You were used to the town . . .'
> 'Well, we had moved from London and we had always lived in a built up area. We never really got to grips with living in the country . . .'
> 'You didn't get to grips with living in the country . . .'
> 'No. That's what I just said!'

The great advantage of the use of reflection, though, is that it allows the client to remain in control of the conversation and allows him or her to take that conversation along the track that he or she chooses. Also, reflection makes sure that the counsellor does not *add* any advice or suggestions to what is going on. Reflection remains one of the most effective aspects of client-centred counselling and is discussed, at length, by Rogers in his work on the topic (Rogers, 1967, 1983).

Checking for understanding

When we are counselling it is important that we understand what the other person is saying and what he or she is talking about. We all tend to invest some words with personal meanings; sometimes we use the wrong word for what we are trying to convey. At other times, we simply let everything pour out at once and it is not clear to the other person what we might mean. The intervention known as checking for understanding refers to the idea that we need to be able to stop occasionally and check what the other person is meaning. If we do *not*, we run the risk of either getting confused or of missing the point.

Two sorts of checking for understanding can be described. First, there is the checking that can take place during a counselling session in order to check exactly what it is that the other person is saying. This is illustrated in the following example:

> 'So I was very worried, really. I mean, I often used to think that I was the only one . . . I found myself wondering what they thought of me. I mean, it was alright at home, but I don't know so much . . . you know . . . people at work and everything. It's not so easy, sometimes . . .'
> 'So you are saying that you were accepted at *home* but not so much at work . . . ?
> 'Yes, everyone at home was fine. Some of the people at work, though . . . they made it clear that they didn't like me.

When people are particularly wound up or excited, they often leave out important bits of information or they run together a range of ideas. In the example, above, the nurse has temporarily stopped the person and asked him to clarify what he is saying. This not only makes sure that the nurse understands the conservation but it also encourages the speaker to become a little more focused.

The second sort of checking for understanding occurs when the counsellor sums up what has been talked about at the end of a session or whenever a natural break occurs. An example of this sort of checking is as follows:

> 'Yes, everyone at home was fine. Some of the people at work, though . . . they made it clear that they didn't like me. Some were downright hostile to me. I don't want to talk about that at the moment. It still feels uncomfortable.'
> 'So let me just sum up, if I can, what we've been talking about so far. First, you feel that you are different to some of your family and to some of the people at work. You also feel that your family can accept you as you are but that the people at work can sometimes be hostile?'
> 'Yes. That and the problem of the job, itself. Yes. That just about sums things up for me at the moment.'

This sort of checking for understanding can be used to close a counselling session. Some people like this approach as a means of rounding things off or of making sure that both parties really have understood each other. Some counsellors, though, find it a little contrived and choose *not* to sum up in this way.

It is arguable that it is sometimes *better* not to summarize what has been talked about in that it can lead to an artificial feeling that everything is somehow rather neat and well packaged. Life is rarely so straightforward and sometimes it pays to leave things a little ragged round the edges. Also, the summing up approach can sometimes also lead to the client packing away his or her problems at the end of the session. While this may sometimes be an important thing to happen, some might argue that it is better for the client to leave the counselling session still thinking about the issues that have been discussed. This sort of counsellor may prefer a rather abrupt ending to the session and might avoid any sort of summary at the end, thus:

> 'Yes, everyone at home was fine. Some of the people at work, though . . . they made it clear that they didn't like me. Some were downright hostile to me. I don't want to talk about that at the moment. It still feels uncomfortable.'
> 'OK. Let's leave it there. It's four o'clock and it's time for us to stop. I'll see you again on Friday and we can discuss things further.'

Think about which approach *you* prefer: the summing up or the abrupt ending. It is important to be clear about one thing here. We are not considering what you would prefer if you were a *client* but what you would prefer as an approach in counselling. As ever, it is important to try to be clear about *what* you do in counselling and *why* you do it.

The time line

We all exist in the present but we all carry our past around with us. No one is very good at predicting the future but we all do it. In counselling, it is useful to work up and down the client's time line. That is to say that it is possible to explore not only the person's present day existence but also their past and their anticipated future.

It is worth paying attention to which aspect of time the client pays most attention to: past, present or future. Then, the skilful counsellor can practise time-switching and help the client to look back, forward or to remain firmly in the present. Some people live in the past because the present is too uncomfortable. Others are always looking forward.

This issue of working with a line can be facilitated at the three levels discussed earlier in this chapter: the feeling level, the thinking level and the concrete level (Table 8.1).

An example of working with the time line in this way is as follows:

> 'We were always unhappy at home. I don't think any of us really liked each other. We used to get very upset about each other for no particular reason.'
> 'What actually happened at home?'
> 'My parents would argue a lot. That would upset me and my brother and we would fight too. Then the whole family would be at it.'

Table 8.1 Questions for working with a time line at the three levels

	Past	*Present*	*Future*
Feeling level	What do you feel about what happened?	What are you feeling at the moment?	How would you like to feel?
Thinking level	What is your theory about what happened?	What are your thoughts about what is happening?	What do you think ought to happen?
Concrete level	What really did happen?	What really is happening?	What do you think will happen?

'What do you think was happening?'
'I think we couldn't bear to face the fact that our parent's marriage was breaking up and we took it out on each other.'
'How do you feel now?'
'What right now?'
'Yes.'
'I've just realized something. I avoid arguments all the time, now. I suppose I'm frightened by them. And yet there is no need to be *now*.'
'There is no need to be frightened any more but arguments still scare you?'
'Yes. That's important. I don't need to be frightened any more. I'm going to remember that.'
'So, the future is going to be a bit different?'
'I think so. I certainly hope so!'

Levels of disclosure

As the counselling relationship deepens and the counsellor and client get to know each other better, so the amount and depth that the client reveals will deepen. The depth of disclosure is a useful barometer of the relationship. If disclosure is not occurring, then the counselling relationship has probably not got very far. A useful device is to think

1st level of disclosure: safe disclosure At this level, only safe issues are disclosed. Disclosures tend to be of the 'everyday' sort: e.g. 'I got up a bit late this morning'; 'I still find work a bit of a problem.'
2nd level of disclosure: disclosure of feelings Here, disclosure is about *feelings*: e.g. 'I feel really angry about what is happening . . .'
3rd level of disclosure: deep disclosure At this level, the client reveals hidden and very personal things: e.g. 'I never really had a childhood'; 'I think I'm homosexual'.

Figure 8.3 Three levels of disclosure

of three levels of disclosure: first, second and third (Figure 8.3) (Cox, 1978).

Everyone discloses at the first level: it is the safe, 'everyday' level. When ever we express something about ourselves to another person in the street or in a shop, we are disclosing at this level. Once we get to know someone a bit better, though, we tend to disclose at the second level more often: the 'feelings' level. Generally, we will only disclose our real feelings to another person if we feel a certain amount of trust with them. The third level is a different level altogether. It is the level of disclosure that we only reach with very close friends or with counsellors or therapists. Third level disclosures are disclosure of deep existential issues: things that really worry us and of which we rarely talk. If you think of three things that you would not like your colleagues to know about, you have identified three areas that would be the subject of third level disclosure.

Third level disclosures are not made easily. Often a person leads up, slowly to making them. Sometimes, the person edges up and then backs away. Here is an example of a 'near' third level disclosure:

> 'There is something else, of course, something I'm not really talking about . . .'
> 'I thought there was . . .'
> 'It's just that, well, you know . . . Oh! It doesn't matter. Let's talk about something else.'

Here, the psychological moment has passed. The person tried to make a third level disclosure but found it impossible. What can you do in counselling when this point is reached? First, it is important not to rush things. The 'I thought there was', intervention may have made the other person feel under pressure. Often, the best intervention as someone heads, painfully, towards third level disclosing is for the counsellor to remain silent. Just sitting and listening is often the approach that helps the other person to disclose. If disclosure does not occur, then it is better if the client is allowed to move on: the disclosure will probably come at a later date. It is usually the case that once someone has made up his or her mind to disclose something important to someone else, then the disclosure *does* take place; the timing is not so important. Certainly it is impossible (and unproductive) to *push* someone towards a particular disclosure.

The level at which disclose takes place depends on a number of things. It depends, at least on:

- How much the client trusts the counsellor
- What the client judges the counsellor will 'make' of the disclosure
- The urgency of the need to disclose
- The atmosphere that exists in the room, and so on.

Counselling rarely stays for very long at the third level. Often, after a deep disclosure, the client returns to fairly light disclosure for the next two or three sessions. It is important that the client does not feel under any pressure, here, and that he or she chooses when and how he or she makes disclosures. The other thing to bear in mind is how the *counsellor* receives such disclosure. Sometimes, the most personal things about another person strike chords in us. We react to third level disclosures according to our own personal history and experience. It is important, after a third level disclosure for the counsellor to think carefully about his or her own feelings. Finally, it is vital to remember that what is a third level disclosure for one person is not for another. The things that the client holds on to might not seem worth holding on to from the counsellor's point of view. It is important not to trivialize or glibly to reassure over third level disclosures. Remember that we are all different. What bothers me may not bother you. Paradoxically, though, it is often true that we *do* share certain common fears and anxieties. Again, it is worth considering how *you* react to someone else telling you something very personal. Table 8.2 identifies some issues that other people have felt to be third level ones. Read through the statements and check the degree to which these would be first, second or third level disclosure if *you* were making them.

Table 8.2 Some third level disclosures

Statement	*1st level disclosure*	*2nd level disclosure*	*3rd level disclosure*
'I'm worried about how much money I spend'			
'I think I have abnormal sexual thoughts'			
'I don't think anyone really likes me'			
'I think I'm gay'			
'I don't like most people in my family'			
'I worry a lot about the way I look'			
'Most people are more intelligent than me'			
'I worry about whether or not I could get Aids'			
'I hated my childhood'			
'I don't deserve to be liked'			

The other issue that arises out of disclosure is the degree to which the *counsellor* should disclose things about him or herself to the client. Jourard (1967) notes that 'disclosure begets disclosure'. If I tell you something personal about myself it is likely that you will tell me something about yourself. This can, of course, be overdone. First, it is possible to overwhelm the client by too much counsellor disclosure. Consider, for example, the following:

Counsellor: 'It may help if you know that I have been divorced, like you. At the time, I went through a very bad phase of depression. It was a very difficult time for me and for the family. Now, how are things for you . . . ?'

Arguably, the counsellor has told too much, too quickly. Second, it is possible to find yourself in a position of what Luft (1967) calls 'paralaction': holding a parallel conversation with the client in which you are both trading experiences but not really allowing each other to expand on what is being said. An example of this is as follows:

'I used to worry, when I was younger, whether or not I was normal. I used to think that I looked odd and that no one would like me.'
'Yes, I know what that's like. I used to be very overweight when I was younger and always thought that no one would ever fancy me because of my weight.'
'I thought I wasn't bright enough. Everyone at school and at college seemed to sail along except me. I was always the one who had to work to finish essays and things.'
'I always thought that I was ugly compared to my friends. They all seemed to be better looking than me . . .'

It would be hard to call this a conversation, it is more an exchanging and comparing of experiences. Certainly, this sort of exchange is not usually a useful one in counselling where the emphasis should be on the *client's* experience. The counsellor may disclose things about him or herself but these are usually kept short and sweet. Sometimes, for example, it is useful to share an experience with the client when you sense that the experience may parallel that of the client. The important thing, though, is to make the disclosure and then move quickly back to the client's world.

'There's something else, as well. I find it a bit hard to discuss this sort of thing. It's . . . the way I look, really . . .'
'It may help you to know that I used to feel really bad about the way I look. I always thought that people were laughing at me . . .'
'That's it! It's stupid, but that's the way I feel! I keep thinking that people don't just ignore me but that they laugh at me as well. I know I'm a bit overweight but I suppose I'm not that bad . . .'
'But you worry about the way other people think about you?'
'Yes. All the time. I suppose I always have. It goes back a long time . . .'

These, then, are issues of disclosure. While disclosure *can* beget disclosure, it is important not to overwhelm or swamp the other person. It is also important not to turn the relationship into a therapeutic one for yourself. Sometimes, excessive disclosure on the part of the counsellor can lead to the client feeling sorry for the counsellor and to worrying about whether or not he or she really should be talking about his or her problems, given that the counsellor is so troubled! This is a less than ideal situation!

Finally, think about how you *handle* other people's disclosure. Some people are embarrassed by other people telling them personal details. Sometimes, too, it is possible to become something of a counselling *voyeur*: the other person's disclosure becomes interesting and the counsellor wants to pursue what is being said more out of nosiness than out of therapeutic intention. Train yourself to notice how much people tend to disclose to you as a matter of everyday course, and what you do when people *do* disclose. In the counselling setting, it is important that third level disclosures are accepted and not met with moralization or disapproval. If they *are*, then it is unlikely that the client will make further third level disclosures.

Putting it all together

The interventions discussed here are never used in isolation. They all go together to make up the skills of the effective counsellor. The passage that follows illustrates how questioning, reflection, empathy building and checking for understanding can work in practice.

'How are you feeling at the moment?'

'I feel pretty worn out . . . sort of uncomfortable. I mean, I feel *physically* all right, but I just feel I have had enough. I feel I have put up with a lot during the past few weeks.'

'You feel you've put up with a lot . . .'

'Well, first of all my husband was ill, then I had the problems at the children's school and now I'm ill myself. It always seems to happen like this.'

'It sounds as though you feel a bit angry with everyone at home.'

'I do! I always have to pick up the pieces. I know it wasn't my husband's fault that he was ill but it's always *me* who has to sort out the children's school.'

'He doesn't give you all that much support over that?'

'He doesn't give me *any*! It's always been the same. He goes to work and I look after the children.'

'Is it just about the children or are there other things?'

'Oh, I don't know. I just feel all stewed up at the moment. I think I tend to blame him when it's all sorts of things. He is very good in other ways. He hasn't been well and everything and the children haven't been all that easy. I suppose . . . they can't find it all that good either. I don't blame them. I don't really blame, him, particularly . . .'

'So it's been difficult because of your husband's illness; the children have been playing up and you feel you haven't had a lot of support from your husband, although you feel he supports you in other ways?'
'Yes, that's about it, I think. I suppose, too, it's something to do with *me* as well. I think *I* have got a bit mixed up . . .'

This extract illustrates the various sorts of interventions discussed and described in the chapter. What it illustrates is the need to pay close attention to what the other person is saying and how important it is to avoid jumping in with either advice or suggested *reasons* for why a person may be feeling the way that they do. In this extract, the client gradually moves from feeling *generally* upset, through the expression of lack of support from her husband, to a feeling of her husband and her children contributing to the disturbance to the hint of other *personal* issues. Arguably, that development of a range of themes would not occur if the counsellor too quickly pounced on *one* thing to take up as a point of discussion. In this early stage of the relationship it is important to keep all possibilities open and to avoid zooming in too quickly on any one issue.

Getting stuck

Like most relationships, the counselling relationship tends to go through peaks and troughs. Indeed, it sometimes seems as though it follows a fairly typical path of intensity followed by inactivity (Table 8.3).

Table 8.3 Typical path of counselling relationship

Start of counselling	*Middle of counselling relationship*		*End of counselling*
High level of activity. At this point, both counsellor and client are enthusiastic, positive and talkative	After initial enthusiasm, the activity levels drop. At this stage, a 'trough' may occur	Renewed activity usually occurs with an increase in energy levels	Towards the end of the relationship, activity lowers again

One reason why this may occur in counselling is that, at the beginning, both counsellor and client are optimistic that change can occur. Both are entering into something new and both hope that things will work out. As the relationship matures, it often becomes clear that there are to be no miracles or magical cures for the problems that are being discussed. Then, a rather more sober period sets in for both parties. Next, having worked through this trough, the relationship typically picks up again and reaches a new peak of enthusiasm and activity as both people get to know each other better and both take a more realistic view of the situation.

Finally, as the relationship comes to an end, the activity level seems to taper off. Perhaps both people are preparing themselves for the termination that is to occur. Perhaps, too, it is better to end the relationship before it becomes totally inactive.

The feeling of getting stuck seems most likely to occur in the middle, trough phase of the relationship. If it does occur, what should the nurse do? A number of possibilities open up.

First, as always, the counsellor can disclose his or her own feelings. Thus it becomes possible for the lull to become, temporarily, the topic of discussion. Sometimes, by disclosing how he or she is feeling, the counsellor moves the relationship on a little and the stuck feeling is resolved.

Alternatively, and again, as always, the client can sit out the stuck phase of the relationship. As ever, it always seems more tempting to do something than to do nothing. And yet such periods can create learning opportunities for the client. Sometimes, it is possible to try to rush in and fix things prematurely. Sometimes the relationship needs a quiet phase in which nothing appears to be happening. Often, quite a lot is happening just below the surface.

Finally, in this shortlist of possibilities, the counsellor can switch tactics and topic of conversation. Having acknowledged that he or she is stuck, he or she moves back from the cul-de-sac and explores new territory. While this is often the most comfortable solution, it may not be in the client's best interest. Sometimes, as noted above, the stuck phase is an important one for the client in that they are wrestling with a variety of thoughts and feelings below the surface.

Most of all, it is important that the stuck phase is not automatically interpreted as the end of the road. New counsellors sometimes feel that getting stuck is a sign of lack of counselling skills and/or ability. While this may sometimes be true, it is equally true that *all* counsellors experience stuck phases at various times.

One other possibility is worth exploring. Sometimes, the stuck phase is induced by the counsellor. This can occur when something that the client is discussing has implications for the counsellor. When the client begins to express difficulties that the counsellor also has, then the counsellor can find him or herself temporarily deskilled. It is as though we are caught in headlights and freeze. Two possibilities occur here. First, the counsellor can accept what is happening and allow the situation to resolve itself. Second, the counsellor can review his or her own problems – with another counsellor, in a group or individually.

This sort of problem highlights the need for all counsellors to develop self-awareness. We often cannot help others without first having some idea of our own problems. That is not to say that we can automatically resolve all our problems. We are all flawed and self-awareness never means problem-free. We can, however, do much to become aware of our own problems and to be prepared to meet them in our clients. After all, we are human too.

Moving on

Finally, the judgement has to be made about when to move on in the relationship. This initial period of exploration naturally leads on to the next: the stage of identifying priorities. Perhaps the most important thing to bear in mind here is that the priorities will emerge. It is not, in the end, up to the counsellor to decide what those priorities are. As the relationship matures, the most important issues become clear to both parties.

Priorities emerge in many different ways. Sometimes, there are one or two particular issues to which the client keeps returning. Then, both parties begin to notice and begin to identify those issues as priorities.

Sometimes, the words that the client uses indicate the sorts of things that may be priorities. We have noted, above, that many people live in a feeling, thinking or concrete domain. The person who constantly uses expressions such as 'I think' and 'I believe that what is going on here is . . .', may have problems in dealing with their feelings. On the other hand, the person who always uses 'feeling words' may have avoided any recourse to systematic problem solving. Alternatively, the 'concrete' person may avoid reflecting at all on his or her life situation and that fact becomes the priority. As we have seen, it often helps if people consider how they feel, how they think and also what actually happens.

Sometimes, the client will acknowledge particular issues as important ones. Then, he or she naturally leads the counselling relationship into the next phase. It is not a question of moving the relationship on, the relationship moves as a natural process.

Above all, it is important not to rush this early phase. It is easy to search for green apples – issues that *appear* to be major problems but which are not identified as such by the client. Mostly, this initial exploratory phase has its own life span. Mostly, the relationship develops steadily until it becomes clear exactly what issues need to be highlighted.

This chapter has examined an important stage of the counselling model: the exploration stage. At this stage, everything is tentative. The client is telling you his or her story. It is not the time for deciding on what should or must be done. All that is important is that you hear as many aspects of the person's story as are possible and that he or she is willing to share with you. I has been suggested that, given time, the true problems will emerge out of that story. There is rarely any need for prompting: most people who want help are only too ready to talk about what is happening to them. Certainly, there is no need for the nurse to develop any sort of theory about the person's life or about that person's problems. The main skill, here, is that of listening: to listen and not to judge or jump to conclusions must be the major aims of this particular stage. In fact, those skills run right the way through the model but are of particular importance in this early stage of the relationship.

Activities for learning this stage

Activity one: review your own skills in this stage. Consider the degree to which you do or do not listen well to other people. Consider, too, the degree to which you tend to form opinions or jump to conclusions about what other people tell you. See whether or not you need to practise the art of standing back a little from what you are hearing and avoid forming too quick a judgement of a person or situation. Think also about your skills in questioning, reflection, empathy building and checking for understanding. Think about the degree to which you use those skills consciously. They need to be used consciously. As with other sorts of skills, it is vital that we *think* about the skills before and as we use them. The temptation is always to saying something like: 'Oh, I recognize all of the things described here. I use these skills all of the time. I don't need to think about them.' The point is, of course, that we *do* need to think about them. If we do not, we run the risk of slipping into well worn patterns of behaviour.

Activity two: write out a dialogue between two people in which one is discussing problems with another. Try to write in examples of all of the sub-skills described in this chapter. Make sure that there are examples of open questions, closed questions, reflection, empathy-building statements and checks for understanding. Try to include examples of thinking questions, feeling questions and concrete questions. This activity is useful for personalizing the skills. In writing down particular sorts of examples that you have invented, you are helping to reinforce learning about them. If you are working with a group of people, have each person read out his or her example and invite other members of the group to comment on the examples.

Activity three: become aware of the interventions that colleagues use when they talk to patients. Do they ask questions? If so, what sort? Do they use reflection and empathy-building statements? What *sort* of interventions seem to be most effective?

Activity four: begin to notice the use of these interventions in a wider context. Notice how dialogue is written in novels. Notice the writing of television plays and see the degree to which the interventions described here are written into various forms of literature and art. Also, notice the use of these interventions in television interviewing: in chat shows and on news programmes. Try to assess the degree to which you feel that television interviewers are skilled in using the various interventions. Notice, too, their use of *silence*. Sometimes, an off camera interviewer will ask a question and then remain totally silent while the person being interviewed struggles to find words and often compromises him or herself in the process! It must be remembered, of course, that this use of silence is not the sort that is used in counselling but it does serve to show the *power* of silence.

Activity five: make a list, for your eyes only, of the things that would be third level disclosures if you talked about them. Then consider what would happen if you *did* discuss them with another person. Consider, too, what *stops* you talking about them.

Questions for reflection and discussion

- What sorts of things distract *you* in counselling?
- Are you a good listener?
- What are the disadvantages of allowing another person to talk things through?

9

Stage four: identifying priorities

Stage One: Meeting the client
Stage Two: Agreeing a contract
Stage Three: Exploring the issues
Stage Four: Identifying priorities
Stage Five: Helping with feelings
Stage Six: Exploring alternatives
Stage Seven: Ending the relationship

At some point, the talking has to stop. At least, the talking *in general terms* has to. There comes a point at which both the client and the counsellor need to consider what the priorities are in the counselling relationship. This is a short chapter but an important one!

Often, these priorities emerge out of the conversation between the two people. There is usually no need to force the issue. Usually, the client comes to realize, over the days or weeks, exactly what the main issues are. Then, it is quite common for him or her to concentrate on those issues automatically. Sometimes, though, things do not go as smoothly as this. Then it is useful to consider other strategies. This chapter looks at some of the ways of helping the client to focus on the important life issues that are troubling him or her. After all, as we have noted, counselling cannot put everything right, nor can it sort out all of a person's problems.

Working at the three levels

As we discussed in the previous chapter, it is useful to get used to working at three levels: the thinking level, the feeling level and the concrete level. In trying to work out priorities, it is also useful to address these three issues. The simplest way of doing this is to address them directly, through questions that work at these levels:

- What do you think are the most important things we have talked about?
- What are the most important feelings for you at the moment?
- What do you think really needs to be done now?

By using these questions, it is possible to help the client to identify important life issues from three different perspectives. A rather more elaborate method of identifying priorities is to use brainstorming.

Brainstorming

The technique known as brainstorming will be familiar to many nurses in training, many nurse educators and those who are involved in management or management training. It is a tool used to generate ideas and then to order priorities. It is simply described.

- First, the client is invited to think of all the issues that have arisen in counselling so far. No issues are to be excluded and the client is encouraged to be imaginative and to mention even the most marginal or seemingly unimportant issues.
- As the client is talking, the counsellor jots down all of the issues raised by the client without leaving any out or ordering them in any way.
- Once the client has brainstormed in this way, both client and counsellor sit with the sheets of jotted down ideas and explore them. It may be possible to put them into an order of priority or it may be possible to group them together according to their similarity.
- Out of this brainstorming will emerge a clear list of important issues that the client will recognize as more pressing than the others. Also, he or she may appreciate some of the things that have already been *clarified* through counselling. Brainstorming is also a useful method for evaluating what has happened so far.

This is a simple but effective method of helping the client to identify issues that are important. As we have noted, it may not be necessary to use such a technique, for very often it will be only too clear what the main issues are. Even if this is true, it is important to stop at some point in the counselling relationship and to consider what needs to be done next and what needs to be talked about further. There is a real danger that counselling can become cosy. That is when the relationship settles down to a comfortable one between the two parties: both are satisfying the immediate needs of the other. On the one hand, the counsellor is acting as a listening ear to the client, who often goes over and over the same ground. On the other hand, the client keeps the counsellor feeling that he or she is doing a good job, merely by being there at all. A cosy collusion between the two people sets in and no progress is made. Whenever you feel that your counselling is jogging along nicely, it is worth asking both you and your client, 'what needs to happen next?'

Developing a priority list

With this idea of progress and forward motion in mind, it is worth considering the keeping of a priorities list. This is a list of the issues that are needy of further work devised by both the client and the counsellor. It is a list that can be drawn up once the previous stages of the counselling model have been worked through and can be kept as a check list by the client. An example of such a check list might be:

- Continue to discuss my relationship with my wife
- Think about how I got on with my parents
- Consider the implications of both of these for my present life circumstances
- Think about whether or not I want to continue in my job
- Think about whether or not I need to do more studying.

Alongside this changing priority list, it is sometimes useful for the client to keep a reflective journal. A reflective journal is a loose-leaf note book kept by the client in which he or she notes down his or her reactions to both counselling and its effects. It is helpful if the client uses a series of headings in order to keep the journal structured. Examples of such headings are:

- What I have been thinking about this week
- What I have been feeling
- What I have been doing this week
- Things that need to be changed
- Things I need to talk about in the next session.

Obviously, the individual client can adapt the headings to suit his or her own preferences. The important thing is that the headings are both useful and encourage a consistent approach to keeping the journal. Without minimal structure, it is easy for most people to forget to fill in the journal, to get bored with it or to decide that it is of less value than they thought. The structure helps to keep up levels of motivation.

A decision needs to be made about whether or not the client will share the contents of the journal with the counsellor. Three possibilities present themselves here:

- The journal remains confidential to the client
- The client discusses issues out of the journal but the counsellor does not read it
- The counsellor reads the journal in full.

A useful approach is to help the client to decide for him or herself which possibility will apply. While it seems an intrusion, for some people, that another person reads their writing, for others it seems a natural progression of a close relationship. The important thing about the reflective journal is that it keeps the relationship focused and allows both client and counsellor to be clear about what the most important issues are in the client's life.

Moving on

Once priorities have been agreed between the counsellor and the client, the counsellor can work towards resolution of the new problems thrown up. It is here that the skills discussed in the previous chapter come into play again:

- Open questions
- Closed questions
- Reflection
- Empathy building
- Checking for understanding.

The relationship, once it has moved on to the question of priorities is likely to have deepened. Third level disclosures are likely to be more common during and after this stage. It is interesting to note that as the levels of disclosure are worked through, one level of disclosure leads to another. It is as though the process of working through one level makes it 'permissible' to work at another. Figure 9.1 illustrates the progression from first level disclosures through to third level disclosures in the course of a counselling conversation.

Sometimes, the process of counselling involves a cyclical process of working: exploring issues in a general way; identifying priorities; working through some of those priorities; exploring issues in a more general way and so on. It is as though a set of priorities are first identified; these are then worked through and out of that working through, the client wants to go back to the broader issues in order to identify a *new* set of priorities. This process of waxing and waning, of opening and closing is characteristic of most counselling relationships. The whole thing is rarely a linear move in one direction: there is usually quite a lot of 'toing and froing'. Often, too, disclosure varies from first to third level and back again.

'It's been an interesting week. I suppose that a lot of things have happend. It's quite difficult to know where to start.'	*1st level disclosures* The client opens the conversation without any 'in depth' disclosure
'I feel a bit uncomfortable. I know what is happening to me and yet I find it difficult to talk about the really serious things. It's as though I'm avoiding things, you know.'	*2nd level disclosures* The client acknowledges the discomfort caused by the underlying problems that need to be talked about. Specifically, she talks about her feelings
'Well, here goes. I realized, this week that I don't want to stay married. I know that's going to cause a lot of people problems and I don't know how it's all going to work out, but I *do* know that I don't want to be married any more. That's the "bottom line", I suppose. That's the thing I've really got to face, painful or not.'	*3rd level disclosures* The client gets down to the priority issues and discloses some very personal and very painful issues

Figure 9.1 Progression from first level disclosures to third level disclosures

What is important is that the whole process does not become static. Sometimes, as we have seen, it is possible for both parties to enjoy the closeness of the relationship and for little progress to be made. Both are satisfying needs in each other. What is needed, at this point, is something of a jolt to move the relationship on. For this purpose, it is sometimes useful for the *counsellor* to keep a journal very much in the style of the one suggested for the client, above. Again, the journal needs to be structured and the counsellor needs to think carefully about where such a journal is kept for it will contain confidential matter. It is usually best if the information in it does not refer directly to the client by name. Keeping a journal of this sort can help the counsellor to review what is happening between him or her and the client and to make sure that the counselling relationship does not become a dead relationship.

Before the resolution of problems occurs, the question of dealing with feelings arises. The issue of feelings and their release can arise at any stage in the counselling relationship. Particularly, though, it can arise during the working out of priorities. Feelings can also run high when partings are being discussed. The next stage of the model is concerned with helping with feelings: not because feelings are *only* expressed at this stage but because, by this stage in the counselling relationship, they are more likely to be expressed.

Activity for learning this stage

Make a list of your own priorities. Spend some time on this and try to work out exactly what it is that you want to do next in your life, what you want to do in the near future and what your future plans are. Then reflect on how you feel about undertaking an exercise of this sort. Do you like long-term plans or are you a person who likes to 'live in the present?' To what degree do your preferences affect how you deal with patient's problems?

Questions for reflection and discussion

- Are you good at identifying priorities in your own life?
- What are the problems for nurses in encouraging patients to make their own decisions?
- To what degree is the nursing profession client-centred?

10

Stage five: helping with feelings

Stage One: Meeting the client
Stage Two: Agreeing a contract
Stage Three: Exploring the issues
Stage Four: Identifying priorities
Stage Five: Helping with feelings
Stage Six: Exploring alternatives
Stage Seven: Ending the relationship

The next stage is that of helping with feelings. The client has sometimes bottled up his or her feelings and this can get in the way of making decisions and of problem solving in counselling. They sit, as it were, under a cloud of emotion which prevents them from thinking clearly and from planning the future.

This chapter explores the issue of feelings. While, in this model, the issue of feelings is raised here, it is fully acknowledged that feelings can emerge at any stage in the counselling relationship. All of the issues discussed in this chapter are applicable to other stages in counselling. The important thing, here, though is the working through of some of the bottled up feelings in order to move on to the next stage: that of exploring alternatives.

Counselling people often means coping with emotions. A considerable part of the process of helping people in counselling is concerned with the emotional or feelings side of the person. In the UK and North American cultures, a great premium is placed on the individual's being able to control feelings and thus overt expression of emotion is often frowned upon. As a result, we learn to bottle up feelings, sometimes from a very early age. In this chapter, we will consider the effects of such suppression of feelings and identify some practical ways of helping people to identify and explore their feelings.

Before going further, a caution has to be noted. It is often noted that people are individual in their responses. It is difficult to make general statements about 'how human beings work'. If we *do* make generalizations, we are likely to find exceptions to them. It should be noted, then, that while the points made in this chapter are true of many people, they are not necessarily true of *all* people. Some people, for example, do not particularly like or want to express strong feelings. There is no need to have an elaborate theory of resistance or denial here, but merely to note that different people do things differently. There should be no hint from the counsellor that people *should* release or face emotions. It is important to pay close attention to the individual's needs and wants. We are all different and *vive la difference!*

Feelings

It is possible to distinguish at least four types of emotion, that are commonly suppressed or bottled up: anger, fear, grief and embarrassment. Heron (1989) suggests that there is a relationship between these feelings and certain expressions of them. Thus, in counselling, anger may be expressed as loud sound, fear as trembling, grief through tears and embarrassment by laughter. It is suggested, too that there is a relationship between those feelings and certain basic human needs.

We all have the need to understand and know what is happening to us. If that knowledge is not forthcoming, we may experience fear. We need, also, to make choices in our lives and if that choice is restricted in certain ways, we may feel anger. Thirdly, we need to experience the expression of love and of being loved. If that love is denied us or taken away from us, we may experience grief. To these basic human needs may be added the need for self-respect and dignity. If such dignity is denied us, we may feel self-conscious and embarrassed. Practical examples of how these relationships work in everyday life and in the counselling relationship may be illustrated as follows:

An 18-year-old girl is attempting to live in an apartment on her own. Her parents, however, insist on visiting her regularly and making suggestions as to how she should decorate the flat. They also regularly buy her articles for it and gradually she senses that she is feeling very uncomfortable and distanced from her parents. In the counselling relationship she discovers that she is very angry: her desire to make choices for herself is continually being eroded by her parents' benevolence.

A 50-year-old man hears that his sister is seriously ill and subsequently, she dies. He feels no emotions except that of feeling frozen and unemotional. During a counselling session he suddenly discovers the need to cry profoundly. As he does so, he realizes that, many years ago, he had decided that crying was not a masculine thing to do. As a result, he blocked off his grief and felt numb, until, within the safety of the counselling relationship, he was able to discover his grief and express it.

A 20-year-old man, discussing his college work, during a counselling session begins to laugh almost uncontrollably. As he does so, he begins to feel the laughter turning to tears. Through his mixed laughter and tears he acknowledges that, 'No one ever took me seriously . . . not at school, at home . . . or anywhere'. His laughter may be an expression of his lack of self-esteem and his tears, the grief he experiences at that lack.

In the last example it may be noted how emotions that are suppressed are rarely only of one sort. Very often, bottled up emotion is a mixture of anger, fear, embarrassment and grief. Often, too, the causes of such blocked emotion are unclear and lost in the history of the person.

What is, perhaps, more important is that the expression of pent-up emotion is often helpful in that it seems to allow the person to be clearer in his thinking once he has expressed it. It is as though the blocked emotion 'gets in the way' and its release acts as a means of helping the person to clarify his thoughts and feelings. It is notable that the suppression of feelings can lead to certain problems in living that may be clearly identified.

The effects of bottling up emotion

What happens if you do bottle up emotion? Most of us are familiar with doing this and before you read further, try to identify some of the ways that bottled up feelings affect you. Also, think about how this sort of bottling up affects some of the people that you live and work with. It is probably true that we tend to bottle up feelings in fairly characteristic ways. For example, I know when I am bottling up some of my feelings because I tend to begin to cut myself off from other people and become rather distant. What do you do?

Physical discomfort and muscular pain

In a way, we all realize the link between the emotions and the body: we all feel physically uncomfortable when we are stressed. Wilhelm Reich, a psychoanalyst with a particular interest in the relationship between emotions and the musculature noted that blocked emotions could become trapped in the body's muscle clusters (Reich, 1949). Thus he noted that anger was frequently 'trapped' in the muscles of the shoulders, grief in muscles surrounding the stomach and fear in the leg muscles. Often, these trapped emotions lead to chronic postural problems. Sometimes, these bottled up feelings are referred to metaphorically by the stressed person: 'I think I'm becoming a pain in the neck.'

Sometimes, the thorough release of the blocked emotion can lead to a freeing up of the muscles and an improved physical appearance. Reich believed in working directly on the muscle clusters in order to bring about emotional release and subsequent freedom from suppression and out of his work was developed a particular type of mind/body therapy, known as 'bioenergetics' (Lowen, 1967; Lowen and Lowen, 1977).

Have a look around at the people you live and work with. Notice their postures, how they stand, how they walk and how they position their shoulders. Then see if you can note the link between 'frozen emotion' of the sort described here, and people's musculature. Hospitals, as examples of large institutions are great places to observe all sorts of rather odd postures! Given that nurses have been generally encouraged to bottle up their feelings it may not be surprising to find examples of chronic posture problems among your colleagues.

In terms of everyday counselling, trapped emotion is sometimes visible in the way that the client holds himself and the skilled nurse can learn to notice tension in the musculature and changes in breathing patterns that may suggest muscular tension. We have noted throughout this book how difficult it is to interpret another person's behaviour. What is important, here, is that such bodily manifestations be used only as a clue to what may be happening in the person. We cannot assume that a person who looks tense, is tense, until he has said that he is.

Nurses will be very familiar with the link between body posture, the musculature and the emotional state of the person. Frequently, if patients and clients can be helped to relax, then their medical and psychological condition may improve more quickly. Those health professionals who deal most directly with the muscle clusters (remedial gymnasts and physiotherapists, for example) will tend to notice physical tension more readily, but all carers can train themselves to observe these important indicators of the emotional status of the person in their care.

Difficulty in decision-making

Decisions are often a problem for many people. Decisions become more difficult when we are bottling up our feelings. This is a frequent side effect of bottled up emotion. It is as though the emotion makes the person uneasy and that uneasiness leads to lack of confidence. As a result, that person finds it difficult to rely on his own resources and may find decision-making difficult. When we are under stress of any sort it is often the case that we feel the need to check decisions with other people. Note any tendency on your part to do this.

Once some of this stress is removed, by talking through problems or by releasing pent up emotions, the decision-making process often becomes easier.

Faulty self-image

When we bottle up feelings, those feelings often have an unpleasant habit of turning against us. Thus, instead of expressing anger towards others, we turn it against ourselves and feel depressed as a result. Or, if we have hung onto unexpressed grief, we turn that grief in on ourselves and experience ourselves as less than we are. Often, in counselling as old resentments or dissatisfactions are expressed, so the person begins to feel better about himself.

I once counselled a student nurse who did not only *believe* that she was ugly, she *knew* that she was, in the same way that she *knew* that she was a student nurse. This was in spite of the fact that everyone who knew her considered her attractive. It was only later, after she had fully expressed some of the resentment she felt for her parents that she came to see herself in a more positive light. It was as though the resentment she felt for her parents was transmuted into resentment for herself. There is another important issue in this example too. What was also difficult for the student was that most people's stock response to her commenting on how ugly she was, was, 'Don't be silly – of course you're not ugly!' Not only did this not help but it tended to reinforce her feelings of ugliness: she merely noted how hopeless other people's judgement was. The important point is to *accept* what the client says as true for them.

Setting unrealistic goals

Tension can lead to further tension. This tension can lead us to set ourselves unreachable targets. It is almost as though we set ourselves up to fail! Sometimes, too, failing is a way of punishing ourselves or it is 'safer' than achieving. Release of tension, through the expression of emotion can sometimes help a person taking a more realistic view of himself and his goal setting.

The development of long-term faulty beliefs

Sometimes, emotion that has been bottled up for a long time can lead to a person's view of the world being coloured in a particular way. He learns that 'people can't be trusted' or 'people always let you down in the end'. It is as though old, painful feelings lead to distortions that become part of that person's world-view. Such long-term distorted beliefs about the world do not change easily, but may be modified as the person comes to release feelings and learns to handle his emotions more effectively.

The 'last straw' syndrome

Sometimes, if emotion is bottled up for a considerable amount of time, a valve blows and the person hits out – either literally or verbally. We have all experienced the problem of storing up anger and taking it out on someone else: a process that is sometimes called 'displacement'. The original object of our anger is now replaced by something or someone else. Again, the talking through of difficulties or the release of pent-up emotion can often help to ensure that the person does not feel the need to explode in this way.

Clearly, no two people react to the bottling up of emotion in the same way. Some people, too, choose not to deal with life events emotionally. It would be curious to argue that there is a 'norm' where emotions are concerned. On the other hand, many people complain of being unable to cope with emotions and if the client perceives there to be a problem in the emotional domain, then that perception may be expressed as a desire to explore his emotional status. It is important, however, that the nurse does not force her particular set of beliefs about feelings and emotions onto the client, but waits to be asked to help.

Often the request for such help is a tacit request: the client talks about difficulty in dealing with emotion and that, in itself, may safely be taken as a request for help. A variety of methods is available to the nurse to help in the exploration of the domain of feelings and these methods will be described. Sometimes, these methods produce catharsis: the expression of strong emotion – tears, anger, fear, laughter. Drawing on the literature on the subject, the following statements may be made about the handling of such emotional release:

- Emotional release is usually self-limiting. If the person is allowed to cry or get angry, that emotion will be expressed and then gradually subside. The supportive nurse will allow it to happen and not become unduly distressed by it. After all, the expression of emotion is a universal human experience.
- Physical support can sometimes be helpful in the form of holding the person's hand or putting an arm round them. Care should be taken, however, that such actions are unambiguous and that the holding of the client is not too tight. A very tight embrace is likely to inhibit the release of emotion. It is worth remembering, also, that not everyone likes or wants physical contact. It is important that the nurse's support is not seen as intrusive by the client.

- Once the person has had a cathartic release they will need time to piece together the insights that they gain from such release. Often all that is needed is that the nurse sits quietly with the client while he occasionally verbalizes what he is thinking. The post-cathartic period can be a very important stage in the counselling process.
- There seems to be a link between the amount we can allow another person to express emotion and the degree to which we can handle our own emotion. This is another reason why the nurse needs self-awareness. To help others explore their feelings we need, first, to explore our own. Many colleges and university departments offer workshops on cathartic work and self-awareness development that can help in both training the nurse to help others and in gaining self-insight.
- Frequent 'cathartic counselling' can be exhausting for the nurse and if she is to avoid 'burnout', she needs to set up a network of support from other colleagues or via a peer support group. We cannot hope constantly to handle other people's emotional release without its taking a toll on us.

A map of the helping process

In helping with feelings, it is useful to have a map. Figure 10.1 charts the stages that can be worked through in the process of helping the client to experience pent-up feelings.

1 Exploring the territory
2 Identifying the feeling
3 Releasing the feeling
4 Reflection after the release
5 Future planning

Figure 10.1 The stages that can be worked through in the process of helping the client to experience pent-up feelings

Exploring the territory

People do not normally identify feelings immediately. In this stage, the client and the counsellor work around emotional issues by talking and reflecting. The strategies below are helpful in working throughout this stage. It should not be rushed for it is up to the client to discover the area(s) of his life that are charged with emotion.

Identifying the feeling

Sometimes, we are not sure of the sorts of feelings that we have about particular situations. For example, it is possible to remember childhood incidents with a feeling of *fear*, only to find, on closer exploration, that the feeling that is *really* under the surface is *anger*. In this stage, having explored the life territory, the feeling slowly emerges. Again, the strategies, below, can help in the process of focusing on the feeling.

Releasing the feeling

The name of this stage speaks for itself. Here, the client expresses the feeling by crying, getting angry, expressing anxiety. All that the counsellor has to do, here, is to allow the expression. Nothing needs to be *done* about it – the client is fully able to work through this stage, given the time and space. And that is the secret of this stage – giving the client the necessary space to express the feeling fully. There is no need for the counsellor to reassure, to attempt to stem the flow or to invite the client to stop. The release of feeling is, arguably, an important part of the therapeutic process.

Reflection after the feeling

Once a person has fully expressed emotion, there is often a quiet period of reflection. It is during this stage that the client has a head full of thoughts and mixed feelings. It is often a period of intense insight and realization. It is as though the release feeling has cleared away a blockage of some sort and the client is better able to see what is or has been going on. Again, all the counsellor needs to do is offer supportive attention and it is important that he or she does not overtalk in this stage. Often, merely sitting quietly, perhaps holding the client's hand, is all that is necessary here.

Future planning

Once the emotion has been released and reflection has occurred, the client is often in a better position to make decisions. In this final stage of the process, the client and counsellor discuss what needs to happen next. Often, the client having released his or her pent up feelings, feels much more able to face the future and is better positioned to make such decisions.

It is with these stages of the process in mind, that we can proceed to a discussion of how to help the client to identify and express his or her feelings.

Methods of helping the client to explore feelings

These are practical methods that can be used in the counselling relationship to help the client to identify, examine, and if required, release emotion. Most of them will be more effective if the nurse has first tried them on herself. This can be done simply by reading through the description of them and then trying them out, in one's mind. Alternatively, they can be tried out with a colleague or friend. Another way of exploring their effectiveness is to use them in a peer support context. All of the following activities should be used gently and thoughtfully and timed to fit in with the client's requirements. There should never be any sense of pushing the client to explore feelings because of a misplaced belief that 'a good cry will do them good!'

Giving permission

Sometimes in counselling, the client tries desperately to hang on to strong feelings and not to express them. As we have seen, this may be due to the cultural norm which suggests that holding on is often better than letting go. Thus a primary method for helping someone to explore his emotions is for the nurse to 'give permission' for the expression of feeling. This can be done simply through acknowledging that, 'It's alright with me if you feel you are going to cry . . .'. In this way the nurse has reassured the client that expression of feelings is acceptable within the relationship. Clearly, a degree of tact is required here. It is important that the client does not feel pushed into expressing feelings that he would rather not express. The 'permission giving' should never be coercive nor should there be an implicit suggestion that 'you must express your feelings!'

Literal description

This refers to inviting the client to go back in his memory to a place that he is, until now, only alluding to and describing that place in some detail. An example of this use of literal description is as follows:

Client: 'I used to get like this at home . . . I used to get very upset . . .'
Nurse: 'Just go back home for a moment . . . describe one of the rooms in the house . . .'
Client: 'The front room faces directly onto the street . . . there is an armchair by the window . . . the T.V. in the corner . . . our dog is laying on the rug . . . it's very quiet . . .'
Nurse: 'What are you feeling right now?'
Client: 'Like I was then . . . angry . . . upset . . .'

The going back to and describing in literal terms of a place that was the scene of an emotional experience can often bring that emotion back. When the nurse has invited the client literally to describe a particular place, she asks him, then, to identify the feeling that emerges from that description. It is important that the description has an 'I am there' quality about it and does not slip into a detached description, such as, 'We lived in a big house which wasn't particularly modern but then my parents didn't like modern houses much . . .'.

Locating and developing a feeling in terms of the body

As we have noted above, very often feelings are accompanied by a physical sensation. It is often helpful to identify that physical experience and to invite the client to exaggerate it, to allow the feeling to 'expand' in order to explore it further. Thus, an example of this approach is as follows:

Nurse: 'How are you feeling at the moment'
Client: 'Slightly anxious.'

Nurse: 'Where, in terms of your body, do you feel the anxiety?'
Client: (rubs stomach): 'Here.'
Nurse: 'Can you increase that feeling in your stomach?'
Client: 'Yes, its spreading up to my chest.'
Nurse: 'And what's happening now?'
Client: 'It reminds me of a long time ago . . . when I first started work . . .'
Nurse: 'What happened there . . . ?'

Again, the original suggestion by the nurse is followed through by a question to elicit how the client is feeling following the suggestion. This gives the client a chance to identify the thoughts that go with the feeling and to explore them further.

Empty chair

Another method of exploring feelings is to invite the client to imagine the feeling that they are experiencing as sitting in a chair, next to them and then have them address the feeling. This can be used in a variety of ways and the next examples show its applications:

Example one:

Client: 'I feel very confused at the moment, I can't seem to sort things out . . .'
Nurse: 'Can you imagine your confusion sitting in that chair over there . . . what does it look like?'
Client: 'It looks like a great big ball of wool . . . how odd!'
Nurse: 'If you could speak to your confusion, what would you say to it?'
Client: 'I wish I could sort you out!'
Nurse: 'And what's your confusion saying back to you?'
Client: 'I'm glad you don't sort me out – I stop you from having to make any decisions!'
Nurse: 'And what do you make of that?'
Client: 'I suppose that could be true . . . the longer I stay confused, the less I have to make decisions about my family . . .'

Example two:

Nurse: 'How are you feeling about the people you work with . . . you said you found it quite difficult to get on with them . . .'
Client: 'Yes, it's still difficult, especially my boss'
Nurse: 'Imagine your boss is sitting in that chair over there . . . how does that feel?'
Client: 'Uncomfortable! He's angry with me!'

Nurse: 'What would you like to say to him?'
Client: 'Why do I always feel scared of you . . . why do you make me feel uncomfortable?'
Nurse: 'And what does he say?'
Client: 'I don't! It's you that feels uncomfortable, not me . . . You make yourself uncomfortable . . . (to the nurse) He's right! I do make myself uncomfortable but I use him as an excuse . . .'

The 'empty chair' can be used in a variety of ways to set up a dialogue between either the client and his feelings or between the client and a person that the client talks 'about'. It offers a very direct way of exploring relationships and feelings and deals directly with he issue of projection – the tendency we have to see qualities in others that are, in fact, our own. Using the empty chair technique can bring to light those projections and allow the client to see them for what they are. Other applications of this method are described in detail by Perls (1969).

Paradoxical interventions

A paradoxical counselling intervention may be described (rather clumsily) as offering exactly the wrong intervention at exactly the right time. It is as though the counsellor 'wrong foots' the client and encourages the client to *continue* the way they feel rather than to counteract it. Consider, for example, the following exchange:

'I'm really anxious at the moment, I feel so anxious I think I'm going to cry . . .'
'Can you get a little *more* anxious . . . ?'

This is one example of the paradoxical approach. What would normally happen is that the nurse would try to reassure the anxious person. In the paradoxical approach, and with careful timing and tact, the nurse encourages the feeling being expressed. The outcome can be variable but what often happens is either that the person laughs and some of the anxiety is dispelled through the harmless emotion of laughter or, alternatively, the anxiety does increase and the person bursts into tears.

The paradoxical approach is not for every counsellor nor for every client. It can be very effective if used wisely and with skill. Victor Frankl (1975) has written widely about this contradictory approach to counselling and the interested reader is recommended to read his work.

Contradiction

It is sometimes helpful if the client is asked to contradict a statement that they make, especially when that statement contains some ambiguity. An example of this approach is as follows:

> **Client**: (looking at the floor) 'I've sorted everything out now: everything's OK.'
> **Nurse**: 'Try contradicting what you've just said . . .'
> **Client**: 'Everything's not OK . . . Everything isn't sorted out' . . . (laughs) . . . that's true, of course . . . there's a lot more to sort out yet . . .'

Exaggerated emotions

This is an odd one. Sometimes, when people are talking about difficult situations or difficult people, they use very extravagant language. consider for example, the following descriptions:

> 'He's the kindest person I have ever met. I was really surprised that he acted like this . . .'
> 'I can't think of anyone who means as much as he does to me . . .'
> 'I love both of them very much indeed and couldn't imagine meeting anyone else like them . . .'

Sometimes, this rather dramatic use of language is covering up other sorts of feelings (often, negative ones). When you sense that this may be the case, it is sometimes helpful gently to challenge the statement. An example would be as follows:

> 'He is the kindest person I have ever met. I was really surprised that he acted like this . . .'
> 'It came as a complete shock to you? You really didn't imagine he could be like this . . . ?'
> (laughs) 'Well . . . I suppose . . . now I think of it he was *sometimes* difficult to live with . . . Come to think of it, sometimes he made me *really angry*'.

Mobilization of body energy

Developing the theme discussed above regarding the idea that emotions can be trapped within the body's musculature, it is sometimes helpful for the nurse to suggest to the client that he stretches, or takes some very deep breaths. In the process, the client may become aware of tensions that are trapped in his body and begin to recognize and identify those tensions. This, in turn, can lead to the client talking about and expressing some of those tensions. This is particularly helpful if, during the counselling conversation, the client becomes less and less mobile and adopts a particularly hunched or curled-up position in his chair. The invitation to stretch serves almost as a contradiction to the body position being adopted by the client at that time.

Exploring fantasy

We often set, fairly arbitrary, limits on what we think we can and cannot do. When a client seems to be doing this it is sometimes helpful to explore what may happen if this limit was broken. An example of this is as follows:

> **Client**: 'I'd like to be able to go abroad for a change, I never seem to go very far on holiday.'
> **Nurse**: 'What stops you?'
> **Client**: 'Flying, I suppose . . .'
> **Nurse**: 'What's the worst thing about flying?'
> **Client**: 'I get very anxious?'
> **Nurse**: 'And what happens if you get very anxious?'
> **Client** 'Nothing really! I just get anxious!'
> **Nurse**: 'So nothing terrible can happen if you allow yourself to get anxious?'
> **Client**: 'No, not really . . . I hadn't thought about it like that before . . .'

Rehearsal

Sometimes the anticipation of a coming event or situation is anxiety provoking. The nurse can usefully help the client to explore a range of feelings by rehearsing with him a future event. Thus the client who is anticipating a forthcoming interview may be helped by having the nurse act the role of an interviewer, with a subsequent discussion afterwards. The client who wants to develop the assertive behaviour to enable him to challenge his boss may benefit from role-playing the situation in the counselling session. In each case, it is important that both client and nurse 'get into role' and that the session does not just become a discussion of what may or may not happen. The actual playing through and rehearsal of a situation is nearly always more powerful than a discussion of it.

Alberti and Emmons (1982) offer some useful suggestions about how to set up role-plays and exercises for developing assertive behaviour and Wilkinson and Canter (1982) describe some useful approaches to developing socially skilled behaviour. Often, if the client can practise effective behaviour, then the appropriate thoughts and feelings can accompany that behaviour. The novelist, Kurt Vonnegut, wryly commented that: 'We are what we pretend to be – so take care what you pretend to be' (Vonnegut, 1968). Sometimes, the first stage in changing is trying out a new pattern of behaviour or a new way of thinking and feeling. Practice, therefore, is invaluable.

This approach develops from the idea that what we think influences what we feel and do. If our thinking is restrictive, we may begin to feel that we can or cannot do certain things. Sometimes having these barriers to feeling and doing challenged can free a person to think, feel and act differently.

These methods of exploring feelings can be used alongside the client-centred interventions described in a previous chapter. They need to be practised in order that the nurse feels confident in using them and the means to developing the skills involved are identified in the final chapter of this book. The domain of feelings is one that is frequently addressed in counselling. Counselling people who want to explore feelings takes time and cannot be rushed. Also, the development and use of the various skills described here is not the whole of the issue. Nurses working with motions need, also, to have developed the personal qualities that have been described, elsewhere: warmth, genuineness, empathic understanding and unconditional positive regard. Emotional counselling can never be a mechanical process but is one that touches the lives of both client and nurse.

Art and nature

Sometimes, and for some people, art and nature help in the release of feelings. Obviously, different people feel differently about these things but it is worth considering whether or not your client may appreciate listening to a particular piece of music or reading a particular poem. The point needs to be made that the music or poem must be chosen by the client. There is nothing worse than discovering that what we think is moving is not necessarily moving to another person. Our record or cassette collections reflect our taste and emotions: we cannot expect other people automatically to like them.

Sometimes, too, walking with the client in the open air, in a wood, by the sea or on the downs can help in the expression and release of feelings. Counselling does not have to take place indoors nor in the office. Clearly, there may be practical limitations to the amount of mobility either or both of you may have but think about the possibilities of moving out into the open if the client feels restricted by the environment.

A summary of the process of helping with feelings

It is helpful to review the whole process of the question of feelings. In Table 10.1 various stages in the process are identified alongside the appropriate counsellor responses. It reflects the stages from the 'Map' shown in Figure 10.1.

Table 10.1 highlights the various phases that the client is likely to work through when dealing with emotions. A particularly important point is that contained in item 4. After catharsis (or emotional release) has occurred, there is usually a natural reflective period during which the client may have all sorts of new insights about what has been happening to him or her.

It is as thought the emotional cloud has lifted and the client is able to see more clearly. During this period, the counsellor needs do very little except support the client. Certainly there is no need for intensive questioning or talking. In this phase, the client is doing the work and is often achieving more than will be the case in any other part of the counselling relationship.

The client's feelings or your feelings?

What is really important is that you distinguish between the *client's* feelings and *your* feelings. Often, if the client begins to talk about something that you find emotionally disturbing, you will find that your own feelings begin to surface. The danger, here, is that you will assume that what is causing *you* distress, is also distressing for the client. It is an assumption that is often not supported. We are not all moved by the same sorts of things. We do not all get upset by the same sets of circumstances. We have all lived different lives and carry

Table 10.1 The process of helping with feelings

Client status	*Counsellor role*
1 Client feels 'blocked' and unable to move on in the counselling relationship. He or she acknowledges that he or she cannot express feelings	1 The counsellor listens and accepts and does not offer advice or prescription. Rather, he or she helps the client to focus on feelings
2 The client begins to experience some of his or her feelings. Conversation changes very specifically from 'I sometimes get very upset . . .' to 'I *am* very upset . . .'	2 The counsellor listens and encourages the expression of emotion
3 The client may experience catharsis: the expression of tears, anger, fear or laughter	3 The counsellor is supportive and allows full expression
4 The client sits and reflects quietly, following the cathartic release. This may be a lengthy process and need not be rushed	4 No interventions are necessary. The client is working through a natural process. The counsellor remains supportive and quiet
5 The client feels refreshed and more able to move on to identifying priorities and to solving problems	5 The counsellor takes his or her cues from the client and allows the relationship to move on at the client's pace

around with us different sets of 'emotional baggage'. If you find yourself upset by what the client is saying, you can do one of two things.

First, you can ask the client what he or she is feeling and then you can believe them when they tell you. Second, you can take a moment to 'look inside' and to check what is distressing you. Often, when you do this, you will find that it is something in your own life that is generating the distress. It is not that you are becoming upset on behalf of the client. These two checks can, of course, be used together. They can be helpful in separating out the client's feelings from your own.

Remember: you are there for the client. You can work on your own problems and your own feelings on another occasion. The counselling relationship is not the vehicle for sorting yourself out.

Activity for learning this stage

Read through the following list of feelings. Then underline the ones you feel comfortable with: (a) in yourself, and (b) when other people express them.

- Affection
- Anger
- Anxiety
- Amusement
- Appreciation
- Confidence
- Contentedness
- Disgust
- Delight
- Energy
- Enjoyment
- Enthusiasm
- Fear
- Hate
- Love
- Misery
- Peace
- Upset
- Surprise
- Worry.

Questions for reflection and discussion

- How well do you cope with your own feelings?
- What do you do when someone starts to cry?
- Are there disadvantages to encouraging people to express emotion?

11

Stage six: exploring alternatives

Stage One: Meeting the client
Stage Two: Agreeing a contract
Stage Three: Exploring the issues
Stage Four: Identifying priorities
Stage Five: Helping with feelings
Stage Six: Exploring alternatives
Stage Seven: Ending the relationship

The two previous chapters discussed two of the most therapeutic aspects of counselling: focusing the problem and helping with feelings. Often, the main issue in counselling is for the client to find out exactly what the problem is. It is surprising how much we all can fool ourselves about what is wrong. We tend to go all round the houses but refuse to face ourselves. One of the main functions of the counsellor is to help the other person to face him or herself and then to cope with the feelings that accompany that.

Finally, though, the client also has to *do* something. It is one thing to accept, at a thinking and feeling level, what is wrong. It is another to do something about it. Not all problems, of course, can 'have something done about them'. If you are terminally ill or your social situation is such that it is impossible for you to change the way that you live, then *acceptance* is the action that is taken. Sometimes, too, counselling is about helping the client to accept rather than actively to *do*. At other times, though, it is about helping the client to decide upon a course of action and to accompany that person, a little, while they take that course of action. Often, though, the work that is done in this stage is done by the client, away from the counselling situation. Sometimes, too, the *doing* comes about as a result of focusing the issues and coping with feelings: the relief that comes from the previous two stages is enough to help the client to change his or her behaviour.

Exploring possible alternatives

How, then, do you and the client decide on what is to be done? Sometimes, this stage is fairly simple – the question is asked: 'What has to happen now?' and the client identifies a course of action. Sometimes, though, the client is still confused or uncertain about what needs to be done. Sometimes, too, the client is very reluctant to *do* anything. As we have noted earlier in this book, it is often easier to remain in the domain of thinking and feeling: doing is sometimes more difficult. For other people, the issue is that they want *things* to change but they do not want to change themselves. It is as though the client is saying 'show me how I can make my situation change but make it so that *I* do not change'. The truth seems to be, though, that if we want change to occur in our lives then we must also change.

Problem solving

Formal problem solving is sometimes useful here. The stages of a problem solving cycle are these:

- Identification of the problem
- Generation of all possible solutions
- Selection of a particular solution
- Institution of the particular solution
- Evaluating the effectiveness of the solution.

In terms of the counselling relationship, the first stage of this problem-solving cycle has already been completed in stage four of this model. In that stage, the client was encouraged to identify the crux of

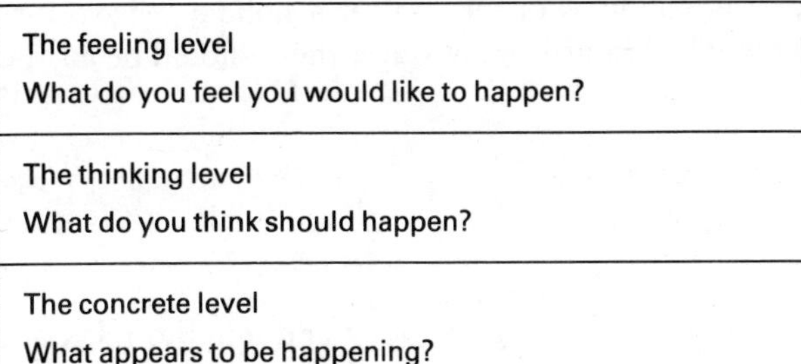

Figure 11.1 Problem solving

his or her problems. It is time, then, to move on to the second stage – the generation of possible solutions. Again, the skills involved in doing this have been described in an earlier chapter: the process of *brainstorming* is the most useful way of generating a wide range of possible solutions. It is helpful if all sorts of solutions are generated: the more extreme, the better. For example, a client who discovers that she no longer wants to return to her husband might generate the following list of 'brainstormed' solutions. Some seem feasible but others, at first sight, seem highly unlikely:

- Never go home
- Walk out, once I'm home
- Disappear
- Talk to husband
- Talk to family as a group
- Talk to the children on their own
- Go and see a RELATE counsellor
- Take a long holiday
- Go to sea
- Go to stay with my sister in Australia
- Have an affair
- Go home and argue
- Go home and stay.

The list could no doubt be added to. In the end, certain options seem to rule themselves out but the *process* of generating *unlikely* as well as *likely* solutions often opens up other possibilities. For example, the 'go to sea' option seems to be a reasonably unlikely option but thinking about it may raise possibilities of moving, of a holiday, of working overseas and so on. The brainstorming stage, then, should be a slow, open-ended one.

Focusing

This is a simple process of allowing the body and mind to relax and thus enabling a 'felt sense' of one's problems to emerge. The process allows for a natural process of problem solving to occur. The focusing approach outlined here is based on that described by Eugene Gendlin (Gendlin, 1981; Hales-Tooke, 1989). Gendlin argued that focusing encapsulated the essence of the counselling process: it enables the person to solve problems at a deep level but more quickly than is usual with more formal counselling methods.

Focusing can be used in a variety of ways by both the nurse as counsellor and by the nurse for her own use. Here, it is described as a number of simple stages. It is probably best if you try it out yourself before you use it to help others.

1 Sit quietly and breath deeply for a while. Allow yourself to relax completely. Notice the thoughts and feelings that flood into your mind. Slowly, but without worrying too much, identify each one.
2 Having identified each thought or feeling that comes drifting into your mind, find some way of 'packaging up' each of those thoughts and feelings. Some people find it easiest to imagine actually wrapping each issue up into a parcel. Others imagine putting each item into a box and sealing it with tape. However you do it, allow each thought or feeling to be packaged in some way. Then imagine those thoughts or feelings, in their packages, laid out in front of you. Notice, too, the sense of calmness that goes with having packaged up your thoughts and feelings in this way.
3 Now, in your mind, look around at those packages and notice which one of them is calling for attention. Sometimes there will be more than one but try to focus on the one that is *most* in need.
4 Now unpack that one particular issue and allow it some breathing space. Do not immediately put a name to it or rush to sort it out. Instead, allow yourself to be immersed in that particular issue.
5 When you have spent some minutes immersing yourself in this way, ask yourself: 'what is the *feeling* that goes with this issue?' Do not

rush to put a label to it – try one or two labels, tentatively at first. Allow the label to emerge out of the issue. This feeling that emerges in this way can be described as the 'felt sense' of the issue or problem.

6 Once you have identified this 'felt sense' in this way, allow yourself to explore it for a while. What other feelings go with it? What other thoughts do you associate with it? And so on.
7 Once you have explored the felt sense in this way, ask yourself, 'What is the *nub of all this*?' As you ask this, allow the real issue behind all your thoughts to emerge and to surface. Often, the nub or bottom line is quite a different issue to the one that you started with.
8 When you have identified the nub or the crux of the issue, allow yourself to explore that a little. Then identify what it is you have to do next. Do not do this too hastily. Again, try out a number of solutions before you settle on what has to be done. Do not rush to make up your mind but rather let the next step emerge of its own accord. Once you have identified the next thing that you have to do, acknowledge to yourself that this is the end of the activity for the time being.
9 Allow yourself some more deep breaths. Relax quietly and then rouse yourself gently.

Recording counselling

At this point, it is important to consider whether of not you will *record* your counselling sessions. What is discussed in this section is of relevance to any part of the counselling relationship.

To record or not to record? Before we discuss a method of recording counselling, it is worth considering whether sessions should be recorded at all.

First, the advantages of recording:

- A series of records allow you to check progress: yours as a counsellor and the client's in terms of the effectiveness of the relationship
- Records allow you to review what has happened between you and the client
- Records enable other people to see what you have been doing in your counselling sessions.

Now, the disadvantages:

- Records can give a false sense of what is happening in a person's life. If you read a record card from last week, just before you counsel, the danger is that you will expect the client's life to pick up from that point when you meet him or her. In fact, though, the client has lived another week since you made your record. A lot can happen in a week
- The real problem and potential disadvantage is the issue of confidentiality. If you make a record, you make a formal document which (presumably) is the property of the hospital or health district. This raises a number of subsequent questions. How *much* do you record of what someone said? Who will see the records? Can you write *anonymous* records that do not name the client?

The question of whether or not you keep records of counselling is far from simple. You need to think long and hard about the issue, discuss it with your senior nurses and lecturers and then make a decision. It may, of course, be possible to write notes in other documents relating to the patient's care as a contrast to keeping separate 'counselling notes.' If you *do* decide to keep notes, Figure 11.2 is one example of the sort of note-cards you can keep. The card identifies the key issues that you discussed during your session. There is space to make notes about the client's expressed feelings and thoughts. There is also a space for writing in what has been agreed as an action plan. This is of particular relevance to decisions made during the current stage of the model of counselling. Finally, there is a space for you to jot down your own comments about the session. It is useful, here, to note down any hunches or intuitions that you have about the client. These are comments that are not necessarily based on what the client has *said* but more on what you have picked up from the client. Carl Rogers noted that he felt himself to be doing his best counselling when he learned to rely on his intuitions (Rogers, 1967).

Recording counselling sessions on computer

More and more health authorities and individuals are using computers to record data. Another option is to keep computerized records of counselling sessions using one of the many database programs such as *paradox*, *dBase*, *PC File* or similar. If such records are kept, it is essential that you check whether or not you are allowed to keep such records under the Data Protection Act, within your health authority.

Name	Unit/Ward
Date	Time
Key Issues	
Feelings Expressed	
Thoughts Discussed	
Action agreed	
Comments	Next Meeting

Figure 11.2 Counselling note-card

The database system gives you much more flexibility for recording your sessions and Figure 11.3 illustrates one possible layout of fields for such a database set up. A separate directory is required for each client and then each record in that directory records the number of the session, the date of the meeting, the topics discussed and so forth. Searching the database will allow you to establish the degree to which progress in counselling has or has not been made. The database format illustrated in Figure 11.3 can be used on any personal computer or network system.

Session number	2	Date	21.3.91
Time	3.00 p.m.		
Topic discussed[1]	1,3,4	Mood[2]	
Action to be taken by client	Agrees to talk to husband when he visits this evening.		
Own feelings[3]	Subdued. Difficult to get started today.		
Other comments	Jane is still talking about how depressed she feels, although I sense that she is less so than last week. She has made positive steps to discuss the baby with her family.		

[1] Topics that are regularly discussed by the client are monitored and allocated.
[2] Mood is assessed at each session on a scale from 1–10. 1 = client's lowest mood and 10 = the client's best mood.
[3] Here, the counselling makes a comment about his or her *own* feelings during the session.

Figure 11.3 Suggested database layout

What do *I* do about note taking? Simply this: I do not keep notes. My feeling is that a person changes so much from week to week and from day to day that it is important that I meet that person afresh each time. That means that I rely on my memory to remember the sorts of things that we have discussed in previous sessions and the action that has been agreed by the client. It does not always work and sometimes I regret that I have nothing to refer to in the way of notes. My situation, though, is different from that of many nurses. I work as a lecturer in a university department and do not have to care for up to 30 patients at any given time. That means that I can fairly easily remember the people that I am counselling and keep them separate in my mind. If you are working on a busy ward or in a hectic community setting, it may make more sense to keep notes. One option always presents itself: try out a system of note keeping. If you like it and it proves useful, keep it going. If not, abandon it and return to relying on what comes up in the counselling session.

Alongside the question of whether or not *you* take notes is whether or not to encourage the client to keep a note of sessions. One simple way of doing this is through a form such as is illustrated in Figure 11.4. It asks that the client records the date of the session, some

Please use this card to record the time and date of our next meeting. Once we have met, write your immediate thoughts about the session in the space provided.	
Name:	Unit/Ward:
Date and time of meeting	Thoughts about the meeting
Date and time of meeting	Thoughts about the meeting
Date and time of meeting	Thoughts about the meeting
Date and time of meeting	Thoughts about the meeting

Figure 11.4 Client record card

thoughts about the session and the time of the next meeting. The card thus serves two purposes. It makes sure that the client is sure about the time and date of the next meeting and it also allows him or her to jot down immediate reactions to the session. The time and date issue is a particularly important one. If the counselling session has been an emotional one and the time and date of the next session is agreed at the end of the meeting, it is often easily forgotten by the client. The simple card takes care of two important elements in the structure of the counselling relationship.

Again, not every client nor every nurse as counsellor will find the idea of such a card useful. It is important, though, to think carefully about what helps most. If the appointment card proves to be a useful way of helping both you and the client to remember your meetings, use it.

Taking action

The final part of this penultimate stage of the counselling relationship belongs very much to the client. It is the stage in which the client *acts* as a result of counselling. Just as we noted that the talking had to stop at some point, this becomes particularly important here. For effective counselling must always lead to *action* on the part of the client. The client has to change something about the way he does things or the way he lives. Reflection on this idea will offer evidence of the truth of it. In the end, counselling can *never* just be about talking: action has to occur. And yet this is very often the most difficult part of the whole process. Freud noted about neurotic people that the last things they wanted to lose were their symptoms. Many people want *things* to change without changing themselves. Clearly, though, if life is to change for the client, then the client must do some changing.

It is helpful if the counsellor talks through this 'action' phase of the relationship very carefully with the client and helps to *plan* the course of action. Like all change, it is usually best if life-change takes place slowly and gradually. However, it is important to make sure that it *does* take place! Often, we are quite good at persuading ourselves and other people that we have changed when, in fact, the changes have been so slight as to be unnoticeable and certainly ineffectual. During this phase of action, the counsellor will act as a supportive friend and be prepared to catch the client if he or she fails. Often, too, the client will regress slightly during this change period. Regression refers to the idea that we slip back a little when we are threatened. Given that change is nearly always threatening, it seems reasonable to allow some slippage. In other words, the client may have come a long way in their thinking or feeling, only to slip back a little when they try to *change*. Again, support is required here and the counsellor should allow the regression and not try too hard at making the client return to a more adult status.

This is not yet the time to terminate the counselling relationship, although the end is not far away. It is important that both parties allow the change element to take place successfully before termination is discussed. Anyway, neither client nor counsellor is likely to *want* to talk about ending the relationship at this point: it is far too traumatic for the client and usually a phase in which the counsellor feels very much involved.

One thing often occurs as a result of the client instituting change: other people, around the client, change too. It is rather like a person becoming more assertive. As the assertive person is met by friends and family, they are perceived as 'different' and those friends and family begin to treat the assertive person differently. So it is with action following counselling. That action *must* occur after counselling seems inevitable. It is also inevitable that the client will be perceived differently as he or she changes. Again, it is part of the counsellor's role to support the client during this, often difficult, stage.

Something else happens, too. As the client changes, so does the client–counsellor relationship. After all, the counsellor is one of the important people in the client's life. So it happens that the client, as he or she tries action as a result of counselling, is likely to modify his or her view of the counsellor. Often, it is a case of the counsellor being seen as more 'human' and that often means more flawed. As the client grows in confidence (and this is a gradual process) so to does he or she come to realize that the counsellor is quite an ordinary person after all. Once this happens, the client also comes to realize that he or she may be able to manage without the counsellor's help after all. Then it is apparent that the beginning of the end of the relationship is in sight.

This, as we shall see in the next chapter, can be quite a painful process for the counsellor. The client is changing while the counsellor is not. For weeks the client has been fairly dependent on the counsellor and now he or she is beginning to become much more independent. And yet the counsellor has remained fairly constant. As a result of this changing relationship, it is not uncommon for the *counsellor* to begin to review his or her life-position. There is nothing like another person's changing to cause us to question our own stasis! Handled well, this can be a taking off point for the counsellor as well as for the client. It can be a period on which the counsellor reflects both on his or her relationships and his or her skills. It can also do much to help the counsellor to face up to the fact of the inevitable partings in life. For it is at this stage in the counselling relationship that the question of parting arises.

Aspects of solving life problems

This stage of the model has been about deciding: deciding on priorities; deciding on what action to take; and deciding about whether or not the counselling relationship should continue. Various issues arise here about what helps a person to make such decisions. Another book could be written about what helps and what hinders decision-making but suffice, here, to note some of the aspects that help in solving life-problems. They are offered to spark off discussion and further thought and not as an exhaustive list of factors. Some of the things that help in making life decisions are:

- Being clear about what the problem is
- Being able to express how you feel to another person
- Having self-confidence
- Having a reasonable amount of knowledge to enable you to make decisions
- Not taking *too* long over decision-making
- Feeling secure with other people
- Being able to tackle practical and economical issues as well as personal ones
- Having reasonable physical and mental health or being able to cope with the current status of these
- Having a sense of meaning and purpose
- Being able to undertake further education or training where necessary.

This short list throws up some other issues for nurses as counsellors which have not yet been addressed. Perhaps the most leading and important one is that a person needs a certain amount of *information and knowledge* in order to be able to make some life-decisions. Sometimes, it is important that the counsellor can either impart information or can refer the client on to someone who can. Not all decisions can be client-centred. Sometimes we need help from experts or those who know more about a field of study than we do. Consider, for example, the current state of your up-to-date knowledge in the following fields. Could you usefully and appropriately offer advice in these areas? If not, are you sure to whom you could refer the client for more information?

- AIDS
- Safe sex
- Government benefits
- Selling and buying property
- Getting a divorce
- Specific medical issues
- Questions of mental ill health
- Spiritual matters and questions of religious faith.

In all of these areas (and no doubt many others) it is essential that we know our limits. If we are being asked for specific information in order that the client is able to make life-decisions, then it is vital that the information we offer is correct or we refer on. Before you take up counselling in nursing it is important that you identify your own areas of limitation and find out what other agencies might be at hand to help.

Activity for learning this stage

Write out a list of the areas that you can think of that could come up in a counselling conversation and about which you would have limited knowledge. Next to each item on the list, try to identify one person by name that you could call upon for that information. If necessary, make plans to update your knowledge base. This is particularly important in the field of AIDS advice, which is a constantly changing field.

Questions for reflection and discussion

- To what degree do you use a problem-solving approach in your own life?
- What are the difficult parts of helping someone to make their own decisions?
- What do you need to change in your life?

12

Stage seven: ending the relationship

Stage One: Meeting the client
Stage Two: Agreeing a contract
Stage Three: Exploring the issues
Stage Four: Identifying priorities
Stage Five: Helping with feelings
Stage Six: Exploring alternatives
Stage Seven: Ending the relationship

The end of the relationship. A critical aspect of the whole counselling process. Before considering that final issue, though, we need to consider, first, the ending of individual sessions. For in a way, each counselling session is complete in itself and the way that each parting is dealt with is important.

Ending the session

How do you finish a session? Think, for a moment, about how you finish *any* conversation. Think, too, about how you end a telephone conversation. At some point, in each case, you realize that you have got to stop. You then wait for a convenient pause and then you make some excuse for stopping: you wind down the conversation until you can say goodbye. In those sorts of conversations, both of you are probably aware that the talking is going to stop and both of you are prepared for it. While this is theoretically true in counselling, very often it is the counsellor who has to take the lead in stopping the flow of talk: very often the client will want to carry on talking. The situation is made a little easier by the fact that both counsellor and client are working with the clock. If, as has been suggested in this book, the counsellor has made a contract with the client to start and finish the conversation at particular times, then both parties will be clear about when to stop. In practice, though, it is sometimes more difficult than this.

The experienced counsellor will learn to pay attention to time and will neither underrun nor overrun. Underrunning can sometimes suggest defensiveness on the part of the counsellor. It is as though he or she wants to make sure that nothing too dramatic occurs and somehow closes down the possibility by finishing the session early. On the other hand, the counsellor who persistently overruns may be the 'compulsive helper': the person who feels that they must offer the client every opportunity possible to express him or herself. Neither underrunning nor overrunning is advisable. It is far better to become skilled in finishing on time. The client will feel more secure in the relationship if this happens with regularity. For it is the time limit on the relationship that offers the client security. The best way, then, is to take note of the time, gently draw the client's attention to the fact that there are five more minutes of the session to run and then gently but firmly to finish at the agreed time. One thing to watch for, here, is the client who finishes the session and then hangs back for a further ten minutes after the session has officially finished. For this reason, it is usually helpful to stand up at the agreed time and to *do* something: turn to the appropriate page in a diary, move towards the door, whatever, but do something! The fatal thing is to sit where you are and allow the client to re-establish the conversation. If all this sounds a little drastic it is because finishing, for some people, can be one of the most difficult aspects of counselling.

One very particular problem in closing a session was highlighted by the psychotherapist, Harry Stack Sullivan (1955). He vividly described the problem of the person who, at the end of the session, asks the fatal question, 'have we achieved anything today?' Sullivan, horrified by this particular question, fantasized about arranging his office so that the question could not be asked. He mused that he might one day have his desk in front of a door through which he could pass on exact moment of the end of the therapy hour. In this way, he thought, he might avoid any possibility of the client being able to ask him what had been achieved! The problem of the question, as Sullivan suggests, is that it seems to erase all of the work that has been done during the previous conversation. It is as though the past hour has been for nothing, that nothing has or could have been achieved. I have found the best way to deal with this question is to draw the client's attention to the nihilism contained in it – to tell the client how hopeless a question it is. You will no doubt have your own way of dealing with it but try to avoid the obvious but near fatal response of, 'Well, what do *you* think we've achieved?'

Think carefully, then about how you will close sessions. Try hard to finish on time, not to finish early nor finish late. The possible exception to this rule is if the client is emotionally upset towards the end of the counselling session. But even then, it is quite possible to help the person to compose themselves and still to finish on time. The problem with making an exception for emotional release is that it can act as a trigger for future emotional scenes towards the end of the counselling session. The client comes to associate tears or anger with the end of the conversation and somehow each session seems to end in this way. It may be far more helpful to encourage the release of feeling about half way through any given counselling encounter.

Sometimes, of course, the session is ended by the nature of the nursing shift or span of duty. If you are going off duty then obviously the session has to end. Make sure, though, that you allow a little time between finishing the session and finishing duty. If you time it too closely, you will find yourself more distracted by thoughts of the time than by what the client is saying.

Even more critical, for both parties, is the question of how to end the whole relationship. Ending the counselling relationship can be a major life parting. Like all such partings, emotions are usually mixed at this time. More likely, though, they all work to make both people try actively to avoid the ending. It is to ways of making such an ending that we now turn.

Ending the relationship

It was Bowlby (1975) who suggested the notion of *separation anxiety*. He suggested that if our early experiences of parting (being weaned, going to school and so on) were reasonably well handled, then later partings would also be more comfortable. If, on the other hand, we had painful early separations, then we came to fear partings and tended to become dependent on people for fear that they may leave us. So it may be with counselling. The separation anxiety may exist for either the client or the counsellor or for both. If the latter happens, then it is quite likely that both will collude with each other to ensure that the dreaded parting does not occur too early, if at all. It is possible to read of people who have 'been in therapy' for 20 years or more. Now at least two things could be happening here. First, the person in therapy has very deep seated problems that just cannot be resolved. Second, neither party wants to let go.

How, then, do we let go? Who decides when the counselling relationship should end? Sometimes (but rarely) the whole thing resolves itself easily. The client becomes increasingly independent and then finds that he or she no longer needs to talk things through. Gradually, it becomes obvious that the counselling relationship is breaking up. But let us consider what the implications of this break up are. First, the client is becoming independent. In the first place, he or she was *not* independent: he or she sought out a counsellor with whom problems could be discussed. Independence, on the part of the client, means that the counsellor is not so needed any more. This fact, alone, may be a painful one for both client and counsellor. The client may want to protect the counsellor's feelings and not want to hurt him or her. On the other hand, the counsellor may resent the new independence and seek to find ways to hang on to the client. In playing out these scenes, the counsellor and client are replaying a very familiar scene, almost metaphorically: the *family* scene. What has been described here is a metaphor for what happens in many families. First, the child is dependent upon the mother or father. Then, as the child grows, it becomes increasingly independent. As it does so, it seeks to break away from the family.

It is at this point that it is worth reflecting on your *own* set of family relationships, both past and present. When did you leave home? Did it happen easily or was there something of a struggle? What is your present relationship like with your parents or your children? Reflection on questions like these can help in coming to terms with the ends of counselling relationships. It can be argued that we take our partings with us throughout our lives and replay them, periodically, when relationships end. If we are to cope well with the end of the counselling relationship, we need to review our past histories of partings. For this reason, no particular prescriptions are offered here: merely the exhortation to review the characteristic ways *you* have of finishing relationships. For in the end, the whole aim of the counselling relationship must be to allow the client to regain complete independence of the counsellor. It is as though the counsellor is constantly trying to work him or herself out of a job. While the aim is an heroic one, it is also a painful and even masochistic one.

Handled well, the end of the counselling relationship can be liberating and positive for both parties. Handled badly, it can leave the client feeling rather guilty and leave the counsellor searching for the next relationship: the relationship that will somehow replace the current one. Some counsellors seek in the safety of the counselling relationship another sort of personal relationship that they had never, previously, been able to sustain. For some counsellors, the act of counselling is a sort of replacement therapy: the client stands in as a surrogate son, daughter, friend or lover. In the end, though, counselling on these terms can never be very fulfilling for client or counsellor. Nobody likes to be aware of such a smothering need in the counsellor. Ideally, the counsellor is a person who can take up and let go of relationships easily. In practice, though, and given that we are all human, this is rarely possible. We all need other people, whether we are clients, nurses, counsellors or just people.

Sometimes, the client will mark the end of the relationship symbolically. In a negative sense, this may be through forgetting an appointment, towards the end of the relationship. In the positive sense, it may be through the client bringing the counsellor a small gift to show appreciation. Both examples can tell the counsellor that the relationship is ending (although it has to be said that some therapists construe the forgetting of appointments very seriously and view it as a form of denial of deeper issues). Usually, whether or not there is some form of symbolic behaviour, both parties will begin to acknowledge that the end of the relationship is in view. The final question is this: who should suggest that you part?

As ever, there are few generalities that seem appropriate here. Sometimes, as counsellor, you will find yourself suggesting that within the next few weeks the client should consider when the break will come. Sometimes, you will suggest a date yourself. At other times, and in different relationships, it will be the client who makes these suggestions. Often, it is easier for both parties if the suggestion comes from the *counsellor* rather than the client. First, the client may feel awkward about suggesting a break. Second, by making the suggestion, the counsellor relieves the client of the responsibility of ending. Whatever the case, the break, has, at some point, to be made. When it *is* decided upon, it is usually better that it is made decisively and the agreed date for the last session stuck to. It is rarely helpful to think in terms of one more session. In the end, letting go has to occur for both the client and for the counsellor.

Transference and countertransference

These are two concepts borrowed from the psychodynamic school of psychotherapy. They can sometimes be helpful in explaining some of the problems associated with the ending of the counselling relationship.

Transference refers to the relationship that develops between client and counsellor. As the relationship deepens (so the theory goes), the client becomes more and more dependent on the counsellor. As a result of that dependence, the client is reminded of a much earlier dependence relationship – the mother and child relationship. In transference, then, the client comes to see the counsellor as a good or bad parent figure and associates the counsellor with all things good or bad. Usually, the feelings are positive and this is known as 'positive transference'. Just occasionally, though, they can be all sorts of bad feelings and this is known as 'negative transference'. When positive transference occurs, the client comes to see the counsellor as all-knowing and all-caring: the relationship becomes a particularly close and dependent one. In *psychoanalysis*, analysis is said to be complete when the transference relationship no longer exists and when the client has learnt to become independent again.

Examples of such transference relationships in nursing are numerous. When a patient tells you that, 'you are the only one who *really* understands', or when you find a patient waiting for you to come on duty and worried about when you may be away: in these situations it seems likely that transference has occurred. Equally, it can be said to happen frequently in counselling and, indeed, in life itself. Perhaps, in the end, we have transference relationships with some of our friends and lovers.

When transference occurs, the counsellor is liable to react to it. This is known as 'countertransference': the feelings that the counsellor has for the client. Very often, and particularly if the transference goes unnoticed, the counsellor will merely play out the parent role to the client's dependent child. Again, examples in nursing are not difficult to find: the time when you protect a patient against the doctor or you find yourself taking over a patient from other staff because you feel that you can care for him or her better. Arguably, these are all dependent relationships and are examples of countertransference.

If transference and countertransference are unresolved, not noticed, or prematurely interrupted, the result may be that parting (for both parties) may become very difficult. The client will not want to lose the counsellor and the counsellor will become very protective of the client. The issue of transference needs considering, particularly towards the end of the relationship but, generally, at any time in it if it seems to be becoming an issue. One way of dealing with it is to talk openly about it with the client. Psychodynamic therapists may question this approach because some feel that transference and countertransference are both occurring at an *unconscious* level of the mind: a level that is not subject to our conscious thinking. In practice, though, it is often not difficult to notice that both of you are becoming increasingly involved in the counselling relationship. I have found it useful periodically to stand back from the counselling relationship, with the client, and review how each feels about the other. This acknowledges both transference as it is happening and helps both parties to review the degree of dependence and independence they have.

In the end, both of you *do* have to part. While it is possible to make all sorts of preparations for this parting, the fact is that it can still be painful and difficult. Sometimes, of course, it is neither and the end of the relationship comes at an appropriate stage and as necessary. However it happens, it offers both hope for the future (for the client, particularly, for he or she is illustrating independence) and also a chance for the counsellor to evaluate his or her counselling.

Evaluating your counselling

Again, the three level approach can be used in evaluating counselling. Counselling, as we have seen throughout this book can work on any one of three levels: the thinking level, the feeling level and the concrete level. Figure 12.1 offers some questions at each of the three levels that you might ask yourself once the counselling relationship has stopped.

The feeling level What do you feel about what has happened? What are your feelings at the moment? How do you feel about being a counsellor?
The thinking level What do you think about what has happened? What do you think should happen next? What do you need to *know* in order to become a better counsellor?
The concrete level What has happened? What is happening now? What needs to happen next? What skills do you need in order to function as a *better* counsellor?

Figure 12.1 Evaluating counselling

The three levels of questions can, of course, also be used at *any* stage in the counselling relationship but are particularly effective once the relationship is over and once the pressure to be a counsellor is off.

The end

As with the counselling relationship, so with the model. This chapter has described the final stage in the counselling relationship and has offered practical ideas for working through the ending of it. Partings are rarely easy – particularly when a lot of time and feelings have been invested. Again, part of the learning process about counselling is learning to live with such partings. In this way, the counselling process can be a learning one for the counsellor as well as for the client. For as we learn to cope with partings more effectively, so we learn more about ourselves, our needs and our shortcomings. Whatever else counselling is, it is *always* a humbling process: it always teaches us that we know less than we thought, that human beings are as frail as we are and that, at bottom, we all share similar needs and wants.

Activities for learning this stage

Activity one: review your own life partings. Consider, particularly, how you handled and felt about the following:

- Going to primary school for the first time
- Transferring to secondary school
- Going on holiday for the first time
- Going on holiday on your own for the first time
- Starting a job
- Experiencing a break-up in a relationship
- If it applies, coping with a personal bereavement
- Having a patient that you knew well be discharged
- Experiencing the death of a patient for the first time
- Leaving home
- Changing home
- Changing job
- Changing ward

Activity two: consider how you might handle the following situations towards the end of a counselling relationship:

- The client asks you, at the final meeting, 'What have we achieved in meeting like this?' This may be the most difficult one of all: think about it carefully!
- The client asks you, towards the end of your relationship, 'Can I meet you when I am discharged?'
- The client says to you, 'I feel very attracted to you and I know I shouldn't. I wanted you to know, anyway.'
- The client says to you, 'I know we agreed that I would stop seeing you but I would like to carry on for a few more weeks yet . . .'

Activity three: Sometimes, when the client senses that the counselling relationship is nearly at an end, he or she ends it rather prematurely. Consider how you would handle the following situations:

- The client, having agreed to meet you on a particular day at a particular time, does not turn up
- The client rings you to say that he or she will not be coming to see you again

- The client gets very angry in a counselling session and storms out of the room saying that he or she is not coming back.

Activity four: Rehearse, in your mind, some of the ways that you could handle the ending of a counselling relationship.

Questions for reflection and discussion

- Have there been any difficult 'goodbyes' in your life?
- How do you usually close a conversation?
- To what degree do you feel that nurses deal well with partings?

13

Types of counselling training

This chapter is about training in counselling. While most nurses now receive specific training the interpersonal aspects of patient care, there is still a need for those who will specialize in counselling in nursing to receive training. There is a variety of routes to becoming a skilled counsellor. In the end, though, what counts most is *experience* of counselling. Counselling training can only go so far: in the end, you learn most by doing counselling – you learn about counselling skills, you learn about relationships and you learn about yourself.

As Project 2000 courses develop, the emphasis on interpersonal skills training and on training in counselling skills becomes more pronounced. More and more courses are including counselling skills in their syllabuses. Indeed, it is quite possible that you are using this book as part of a Project 2000 course. However, the essential thrust of all nursing courses is towards developing the 'all round' nurse. Sometimes it is important to go beyond nursing courses to gain specific skills. Some these courses are also discussed in this chapter.

Short workshops and courses

A popular means of developing counselling skills is via short workshops and courses. These usually last from one to two days to one or two weeks. They may be run in house by the educational department of the hopsital in which you work or by the college in which you study. Alternatively, many extramural departments of universities and colleges of further and higher education offer short workshops. Sometimes a difficulty arises over obtaining funding to attend such courses and if you plan to take part in one you are advised to negotiate fees and time off as early as possible.

Workshops of this sort are nearly always *skills* based. Often, they take an experiential learning approach towards counselling skills in which you learn those skills by *doing* them. This usually means that the workshops involve a lot of pairs exercises and role play. This approach is probably necessary if you are to learn the very particular skills of counselling. The only problem with a totally skills based approach is that you do not necessarily learn the *theory* behind the skills. While you can get much of this out of books, it is also important to be able to *discuss* the various elements of theory. If you want to continue with counselling, you may be well advised to think about a longer-term course in counselling.

Certificates and diplomas

A number of colleges and university departments offer one year, part-time, certificate courses in counselling or two year, part-time diploma courses. Very often, these two sorts of courses are interlinked. You do the first year for a certificate and a second year for a diploma. Such certificates and diplomas can do two things: they can give you a deeper and broader knowledge and skills base and they can also make you more *credible* as a counsellor. If you are to work as a counsellor or if you want to apply for a job as a counsellor, it is important that you are able to demonstrate that you have the appropriate qualifications.

As with all courses, it is important to shop around. Often, a good way to assess a particular course is to talk to people who have attended it in previous years. Also, you need to find out as much about the course from the college which is offering it. A good course will always be backed up by detailed precourse information. Check, too, the fees for counselling certificate and diploma courses. Counselling is something of a growth industry and some courses can be very expensive. There is no evidence that dearer courses produce more effective counsellors.

Before you start the course you choose, see if there is any recommended pre-course reading and try to make sure that you read any of the books and papers that are recommended. This does not mean that you necessarily have to buy all the books on the list: it is quite possible to order the books through your local library using the Inter-Library Loan scheme. Talk to your Librarian about this but do allow plenty of time for the books to be ordered.

Degrees and master's degrees

If you see your career leading to more and more counselling, you want to teach counselling or you just want to know more about it, you may want to read for a degree in counselling. A number of colleges and universities now offer bachelor's and master's degrees in counselling. A bachelor's degree course is normally a full time one running for three years. A master's degree course usually runs for one year full time or two years part-time. Master's courses normally require that you already have a bachelor's degree or that you can demonstrate prior study to the equivalent of bachelor's degree work.

A bachelor's course will offer you a thorough grounding in all aspects of psychology and theory related to counselling and the appropriate skills. Again, it is important to look around at the different courses and to note whether or not a particular theoretical orientation is offered in the course that you are exploring. Some degrees, for example, are more biased towards a behavioural approach while others favour a psychodynamic approach. Also, it is essential to find out how much of the course is of a *practical* nature and whether or not it will teach the skills that are necessary to practise as a counsellor. After all, a three year, full time commitment is a fairly hefty one.

Master's degrees also vary in their format and their theoretical orientation. Some require that you attend on one day or one evening a week. Others have a block system of education in which you attend for weekends and week-long workshops throughout the year. Such matters are important when you are negotiating funding for money and time with your employer.

A master's programme is usually assessed by course work and through the presentation of a dissertation towards the end of the course. Typically, a dissertation will be a fairly lengthy project of up to 20,000 words in length and a requirement may be that it reports original research that you have carried out. If this is a requirement, you will be allocated a supervisor who will help you to plan and carry out your research. Some master's degrees also have an examination at the end of the first year and many are of a modular design.

A module is a discrete element in a course, led by a module director and is assessed separately from any other module. For example, there may be modules in psychodynamic psychology, Gestalt therapy or humanistic approaches to counselling. Usually, you are able to choose from a range of modules at the beginning of the course and have to do a prescribed number of modules in order to complete your master's degree. Increasingly, the master's degree is being viewed as a higher degree which allows professional people to upgrade and update their skills and knowledge base and is a form of education which is enabling many people who have not got 'first' (or bachelor's) degrees to obtain a degree qualification. It is important to note, though, that they *are* higher degrees : a masters degree normally requires that you are able to submit a high level of written work and are able to demonstrate creative and critical thinking. If you are considering all the options, make sure that a master's degree really is what you want before setting out on this course. If you want, mostly, to develop the necessary skills to work as an effective counsellor, you may find that a certificate or diploma course is more practically orientated. If, however, you want to continue to study the theory behind counselling or you want to move towards the psychotherapeutic domain, then a master's course may be just what you want.

After a first or master's degree, it is quite possible to go further and do original research in counselling for a Master of Philosophy or Doctor of Philosophy degree. In order to register for a Doctor of Philosphy degree you normally have to have a good honours pass at bachelor's level, or a master's degree. Otherwise, you register, first, for a Master of Philosophy degree. If your work progresses satisfactorily, it is usually possible to transfer to the doctoral path at the end of the first year of study. Study for a Master of Philosophy degree usually lasts from between one and four years, while study for a doctorate usually lasts from between two and five years. You need to have a good understanding of research methodology to register for either of these degrees. Many universities and colleges do not offer research methods courses as part of their M.Phil or PhD programmes: you are expected to understand the research methods that you have chosen and be able to work, with the assistance of a supervisor, fairly independently.

Teaching yourself

You cannot learn counselling out of a book. You can to some degree, teach yourself counselling. As was noted at the beginning of this chapter, the important thing in counselling is *experience*. It is one thing to have done a counselling course, it is quite another to become an effective counsellor. The path towards doing that is always via the face-to-face encounter with a range of clients.

One way of teaching yourself is by starting off with a number of weekend workshops, supplementing that with a considerable amount of reading around all aspects of the counselling relationship and then by slowly getting experience in working with people. During the early days it is important that you are supported by colleagues and friends with whom you can discuss the practical and theoretical problems thrown up by counselling relationships. At the same time, of course, it is essential that the anonymity of the client is maintained.

If you do teach yourself in this way, it is also important to decide on ways of keeping yourself up to date. One way is to make sure that you do at least two short workshops a year. In this way, you not only study new methods and theories but you also receive an injection of motivation. Counselling on your own can be a lonely affair and it is good to meet other people who are doing similar work.

Also, it is vital that you continue to monitor your own feelings, thoughts and motives and that you continue to develop your own self-awareness. There are many ways of doing this. First, you can join a support group in the hospital with which you are linked. Second, you can keep a reflective diary in which you record your own development. The following are useful headings for such a diary and they help to lend structure to the process of keeping the diary:

- Personal skills development
- New theory studied
- Report on personal feelings
- Important life events
- New books or papers that I have read
- Progress in counselling
- Plans for the future

If such headings are used, the diary can be filled in on a particular day, once a week. The headings will enable you to trace your growth over a particular period in your personal history. If you work with a support group, you may all want to keep a diary and use the entries for the basis of group discussion. Keeping a diary calls for some determination. Most of us have started a diary at some time during our lives only to find that we get lazy about it or simply forget to fill it in. The reflective diary, however, serves as a particularly useful learning and monitoring tool and is being used in more and more colleges of nursing as a training and self-awareness method.

Supervision

If you do a lot of counselling, it is important to consider what sort of support you are able to get from others. The process of hearing about and talking about other people's problems can be draining on the person who is doing the listening and it is vital to consider whether or not you should have supervision. Hawkins and Shohet (1989) have written an excellent book about all aspects of supervision in the health services and the reader is referred to this for details on how to go about seeking supervision.

Supervision, in this context, means sharing with another person or a group of people, the difficulties and achievements that you have had in counselling. It is possible to set up a supervision relationship with another trained counsellor or, in a group setting, as a support group. The supervision relationship can help in at least the following aspects of working as a counsellor:

- It can help to spread the emotional load
- It can allow the counsellor to identify new issues in the counselling relationship
- It can help the counsellor to guard against burnout or emotional exhaustion
- It can let the counsellor know that he or she is not on her own
- It can offer the counsellor the opportunity to off load and to talk through emotional aspects of the counselling relationship.

Learning to be an effective counsellor is a demanding and rewarding process. By virture of the fact that its subject matter is the human condition, the counsellor, through training, develops self-awareness and considerable self-knowledge. As we have noted a number of times in this book, counselling cannot be learned only through a series of lectures on the subject: in the end, it has to be learned personally and experientially.

Questions for reflection and discussion

- Do you need further training in counselling?
- If you could plan your own training, what sort would you have?
- Should counselling training be part of all nurses' education?

14

Running counselling workshops

This chapter is mostly for people who want to teach counselling skills or who are thinking about the issues involved in running a counselling skills workshop. It will be of interest, though, to people who are trying to develop counselling skills in that it addresses some of the issues that are bound up with the process of teaching and learning counselling.

Teachers of nurses often plan counselling workshops having been on one themselves. Others have had formal training in counselling and want to pass on the skills that they have learned. As always, there is a difference between knowing about a particular field and teaching it. At least three sets of issues are raised when it comes to running counselling courses:

- Educational issues
- Organizational issues
- Personal issues.

Educational Issues

There are very many educational issues to address when it comes to teaching and learning interpersonal and counselling skills. In this section, I want to address some of the leading ones.

Aims

It is important to be clear about the aims of a counselling skills workshop. What are *your* aims? To develop skilled counsellors? To introduce student nurses to counselling skills? To enhance their self-awareness? It is easy, these days, to be dismissive of clear behavioural aims and objectives, but it is vital that the counselling skills facilitator is clear in his or her own mind about the aims of a particular course or workshop. First, if your aims are to produce skilled counsellors, the time needed for such an enterprise is going to be far longer than will be the case if your aim is to introduce counselling skills to students. Second, if *you* are not clear about your aims, it is unlikely that your course or workshop participants will be. Third, many people have already attended introductory workshops. There is nothing worse than going to a workshop expecting to expand your skills to find that the basics are being covered yet again. Clear aims, preferably drawn from the needs and experience of course participants can be all important in avoiding this situation.

Content

What should go into a counselling skills workshop? Too often, workshops are nearly exclusively experiential. That is to say that they draw all of their content from the experience of the participants in the workshop. This can become a closed loop of learning: participants pay attention only to the things that each of them knows; no outside information is given to them. Think carefully about content. My feeling is that it should not *only* depend on what participants bring to the course but should also include fresh content from the facilitator. Think, particularly, about the following aspects of content:

- Definitions of counselling
- Types of counselling
- Theoretical frameworks
- Counselling skills
- Maps of the counselling process
- Procedural issues (starting and ending the relationship etc.)
- Self-assessment of skill levels in the group
- Skills rehearsal
- Evaluation methods

Methods

Having pointed up some of the problems of the experiential workshop, it is important to note that counselling skills can probably *only* be learned experientially. No one ever learned to counsel only by attending lectures. In the end, a good workshop should probably be a balance of both formal theoretical input from the facilitator and lots of time to explore and practise a range of skills. There are many books about how to teach interpersonal and counselling skills and lots of 'cookbooks' of exercises for skills development (see, for example Burnard 1989, 1990). Below, I offer a few examples of some of the ranges of exercises available. There are lots more.

Experiential learning

Experiential learning is the process of learning from personal experience and is a vital part of learning to counsel. Many nursing courses now involve teaching methods that draw on people's personal experience. Examples of experiential learning methods include the following:

- Role play
- Skills rehearsal
- Group activities
- Work in pairs
- Psychodrama.

All of these methods involve a number of characteristics:

- Learning by doing
- Reflection on experience
- Modifying previously held knowledge and beliefs in the light of that reflection
- Relating that new learning to real life.

Reactions to the use of experiential learning methods vary. In a study of the field (Burnard 1991b), I found that many students thought that experiential learning methods could be fun to take part in but also embarrassing. They thought that such methods were useful for learning interpersonal skills and most had had direct experience of them. On the other hand, the tutors in that study tended to favour the use of experiential learning methods more than did the students. They also saw them as useful for learning interpersonal skills and generally recommended their use in nurse training. Many of the students in the study felt that some experiential learning activities were unrealistic and did not anticipate or mimic real life.

The point, here, seems to be that such methods should be introduced cautiously and with the full agreement of workshop or course participants. Sometimes, at the beginning of a course, participants are a little nervous of the training methods which will be used. It is important that dramatic methods such as role play and psychodrama are not used too early in a course. Better, perhaps, to introduce people to the experiential learning approach gradually than to drop them in at the deep end. If people *are* put off experiential learning activities, they tend to stay off them. Given that they remain an important way of helping people to learn counselling skills, this seems a shame. Caution, then, is the keyword. Also, it is important that experiential learning activities deal with real issues: issues that relate directly to nursing care and practice. Otherwise, the accusation of unreality can always be made and, in my experience, *will* be made. Counselling is necessarily a practical activity; the exercises we use to teach it should also be practical.

Evaluation

It is essential to evaluate the effectiveness of your workshop. First, it is useful to get a rule of thumb assessment by asking course or workshop participants to tell you what they did or did not like about the workshop. Other people prefer to use some sort of written evaluation form that they hand out towards the end of a course. The true test of the effectiveness of a workshop, though, is not whether or not people enjoyed it but whether or not it makes a difference to their practice as nurses. I suspect that many people enjoy experiential workshops of different sorts: whether or not they make a profound difference to their nursing practice is quite another issue.

Application to real life

The test, as we have suggested, above, is whether or not counselling skills courses or workshops really make a difference to practice. There are a number of ways in which this can be checked:

- By self-reporting by participants at a follow-up study day
- By the use of journals kept by participants and discussed with the facilitator
- By the facilitator going out and observing participants in the clinical setting after the workshop

- By the facilitator working alongside course participants in the clinical setting in the mentor or supervisor role
- By the facilitator carrying out research into the effectiveness of the workshop.

Clearly, some of these are easier to carry out than others. It is quite a complicated business (although a very rewarding one) to carry out research using observational techniques. On the other hand, the self-reporting at a later, follow-up study day is usually a feasible approach. Whatever method is used, it is essential that some attention is paid to whether or not people change their behaviour as an outcome of a counselling skills workshop. If not, the counselling skills workshop will be remembered as an enjoyable island of experience which bore little relevance to the real world.

Organizational issues

Workshops and courses do not simply happen: they have to be planned – usually well in advance.

Planning the workshop

Think ahead. It is one thing to say that you will run a workshop. It is quite another for one to occur and to be a success. The following are all issues that will have to be addressed if the workshop or course is to work:

- How many people will attend? The minimum for an effective workshop seems to be about six. The maximum is usually about 20. What will you do if only five people turn up on the day?
- What sort of accommodation can you arrange? If you are going to use experiential learning activities, you will need plenty of space. I was once asked to run an experiential workshop at a university and found, when I got there, that I had been booked into a huge lecture theatre and that about 70 people were waiting for me! The moral is think and plan ahead. If you do not ask for a particular sort of accommodation, you cannot expect people to think of these things for you.
- What considerations will you need to make about time? Will people have to travel to your workshop? If so, you may have to start late

and finish early. Will people be expecting to pick up children from school? Again, if so, you will need to think about finishing at about 3.00 pm. If you are using experiential learning activities, the processing of these (the discussion afterwards) takes up lots of time. Do not be tempted to pack too much into each day. On the other hand, do not find yourself with hours of time ahead of you and an unclear plan about what to do with it. Counselling skills workshops should be brisk and dynamic as well as quiet and reflective.

- Can you afford the time? As we have noted, experiential learning activities take time to use. Workshops on counselling skills often run over a two or three-day period. Make sure that your regular work will allow you to concentrate on one workshop for this sort of time.

Running the workshop

Having worked through all the organizational issues that arise before the workshop starts, you are then faced with how to run the workshop itself. There are a number of issues to address here and everyone will deal with them differently. However you deal with them, be clear about them before you start the workshop itself. These issues are:

- How will you *start* the workshop? Creating a comfortable and yet challenging atmosphere is an important aspect of running workshops.
- How much freedom will participants have in deciding on the content of the workshop? If you allow too much flexibility here, the more vocal members of the course will take over. If you do not allow enough flexibility, you run the risk of teaching some people what they know already. You need to think carefully about negotiation.
- How will you organize the material? A useful format is one that starts with a formal theory input from the facilitator and then, increasingly, becomes a climate in which participants undertake learning exercises and activities. It is also quite helpful to punctuate the workshop with short, formal inputs from the facilitator.
- How will you manage the time? It is helpful to deal with issues such as when you break for coffee and for meals, before you start the workshop proper. It is rarely a good idea to freewheel too much. It is usually better to have breaks as milestones or markers in the day.

This helps to give structure and organization on the day. A freewheeling approach can leave some people frustrated and others hungry.

- How will you evaluate the effectiveness of what you do. This issue was addressed in the section before this one. It needs to be considered carefully as part of your workshop strategy.

Personal issues

Running counselling workshops is different to ordinary teaching. The subject matter of such workshops is necessarily personal in nature. If people are to learn counselling skills through reflecting on what they do, this tends to lead to an atmosphere in which people are more frank and open with each other than is the case in ordinary education or training sessions. All this can take its toll on the trainer or facilitator. First, it is important that the person who runs a counselling workshop has a degree of self-awareness. By this I mean that he or she should know something of his or her own emotional strengths and weaknesses. If *anything* may be discussed in a counselling skills workshop, then the facilitator must be prepared for anything. If that anything includes things that are painful for the facilitator, then that person may well find the process of running counselling workshops difficult and an emotional strain.

The net result of running too many emotionally charged workshops should not be underestimated. It is not difficult to experience experiential burnout. Burnout has been widely described as a long-term effect of job-related stress. Experiential burnout is an emotional numbing caused by being involved in too many workshops in which too much emotion is expressed. It is as though the facilitator becomes slightly case hardened or generally finds the thought of another workshop too hard to bear. Sharing experiences of workshops with colleagues can help here as can the development of support groups and support networks for facilitators. Perhaps the best way to avoid experiential burnout, though, is to make sure that you limit the number of counselling workshops that you run and make sure that you vary your teaching/learning style. No one *needs* to run exclusively experiential learning sessions. It is quite possible to intersperse experiential workshops with more formal teaching or lecturing.

Educational skills

In order to facilitate counselling skills workshops, certain facilitation skills are called for. Facilitation differs from teaching in certain, characteristic ways. A short list of the skills of group facilitation would include:

- Skills in encouraging group members to reflect on and make sense of their experience
- Skills in setting up role play, pairs activities and other experiential learning exercises
- Skills in helping people to process such activities
- Skills in handling people's emotions
- Skills in coping with group dynamics
- Skills in dealing with your *own* feelings as they emerge.

Such skills are usually learned on teaching courses or through workshops. They can also be learned through attendance at a range of experiential learning workshops in which such skills are demonstrated. It is often a good idea to model yourself on a particular facilitator until you have had a range of experiences of your own and are able to develop your own style. In the end, of course, you *have* to be yourself. It is no use continuing to emulate a facilitator that you particularly admire for you are not that person. In the end, you have to develop what is usually an amalgam of styles. The point, though, is to continue to develop that style. Just as it is possible to develop experiential burnout, referred to above, through prolonged exposure to too many experiential workshops, so it is possible to develop it by getting into a rut. The facilitator who always uses the same approach, the same activities and teaches the same interpersonal skills is in danger of such burnout. It is important to change your act frequently and develop new and different ways of doing things.

These are some of the issues connected with running courses for developing counselling skills. What follows is a list of questions to address if *you* are thinking of setting up such courses or workshops:

- Are you clear about why you want to run such courses?
- Have you identified a clear need for such courses?
- What would the aims of your course be?
- How long would the course be?

- What experience have you had in using experiential and interactive learning exercises?
- Could you cope with contingencies that might arise through using such activities?
- Are you clear about how to use the available time?
- Are you clear about the educational principles involved?
- Are you happy that you can offer a fairly comprehensive *range* of counselling skills exercises?
- How much counselling experience have you had?
- Are you continuing your own growth and development?
- Are you continuing to meet your own education wants and needs?

Finally, in this chapter, some examples of activities that can be used in counselling courses are offered. This is by no means an exhaustive presentation of the activities that can be used, but the examples here can all be *modified* by the facilitator to reflect the needs and wants of the group. An important part of being a facilitator is being able to be flexible and to respond to the changing needs of workshop participants. The activities are presented under a series of headings that cover almost all aspects of a counselling skills course:

- Activities for starting a counselling skills workshop
- Activities to encourage thinking about counselling in nursing
- Activities which develop listening skills
- Activities which encourage client-centred counselling skills
- Activities to use at the end of learning session
- Activities for ending a counselling workshop.

Activities for starting a counselling skills workshop

Activity one: Perhaps the most straightforward way of encouraging people to talk and to talk to each other is through the use of a round. A round, as it suggests, is a process through which each person in turn says something about themselves to the rest of the group. An introductory round can involve each person in saying the following:

- Their name (and the name they prefer to be known by)
- Their job
- Something about themselves which is not related to work.

Various modifications to this basic format can be suggested. First, after each person has spoken, it is possible to suggest that the rest of the group feel free to ask questions of that person. This can encourage early group participation. Second, the *subject* of the round can be changed to reflect different facilitator styles or different groups. For example, the subject of the round could be any one of the following:

- How you feel about being here
- What you hope to get from the workshop
- Your experience of counselling to date
- How you feel at this moment
- Your name, age and where you live.

The round is a very flexible activity which can easily be modified and used at various points during the life of a workshop.

Activity two: a different starting activity is to invite group participants to pair off and interview each other for about 10 minutes. After 10 minutes have passed, the larger group reconvenes and each person introduces the other person to the group. Again, this can be done as a formal round or, after each person has been introduced, group members may be invited to ask questions. Like the round, the pairs interview is an adaptable activity which can be used for a variety of purposes during the counselling skills workshop.

Activity three: with younger and fairly extrovert groups, the *icebreaker* is an opening option. Icebreakers offer people a chance to start a workshop informally, with some activity and with the opportunity for everyone to be involved in doing something. Here are three examples of icebreakers:

- Group participants are invited to stand up and mill around the room. At a signal from the facilitator, people stop and introduce themselves to the people closest to them. The aim should be to continue milling and stopping until everyone has met everyone.
- Group participants stand and move around the room, hugging every other participant in turn. This is obviously a fairly intimate icebreaker and probably not for the uninitiated!
- Group participants sit in a circle. First, each person in turn says their name. Then, the facilitator throws a cushion to one of the participants, saying their name as he or she does so. The person

who catches the cushion then throws it to someone else, naming him or her in the process. This throwing and naming is continued until everyone in the room is confident that he or she knows the name of everyone else.

Activities to encourage thinking about counselling in nursing

Once the workshop has started and the facilitator has dealt with domestic issues such as breaks, timetable of events and so forth and before a formal theory input is offered, it is often useful to invite participants to reflect on what they think counselling is.

Activity four: participants are invited to pair off. One of each pair is nominated A and the other B. A then talks to B for five minutes, without B responding in any way but to listen on the topic, 'What I believe counselling to be.' After five minutes, roles are reversed and B talks to A while A only listens. It is usually necessary to underline the fact that the exercise is not a conversation but that it is a listening exercise as much as one that can help to clarify concepts and ideas. After a further five minutes, the group reconvenes and participants share their experiences.

This format is a particularly versatile one. A wide range of themes can be used for exploration in the pairs format. A short list of such themes includes:

- What are counselling skills?
- How can counselling be used in nursing?
- How can you teach counselling?
- What are the problems in nurses' counselling?
- What are you like as a counsellor?
- What do you need to learn from this workshop?
- What are your feelings about being here?

Activity five: an alternative to the pairs format is the group brainstorm. The process of brainstorming has already been described in an earlier chapter. The procedure for group brainstorming is as follows:

- The facilitator has a blank flip-chart pad or a clean white or blackboard in front of the group which has on it the heading for the brainstorming session. Examples of appropriate headings are the same as those themes identified above as suitable for using pairs

- The facilitator then invites group members to call out words and phrases that they associate with the theme
- All words and phrases are written down by the facilitator who makes no attempt to edit what is said nor attempts to correct or modify any offering. The aim is to collate as many different sorts of ideas as possible
- After about 15 minutes, the facilitator helps the group to sort the ideas and themes under different headings. An example of such sorting is illustrated in Figure 14.1
- After the brainstorming activity, the group discusses the themes and ideas that are in front of them.

This sort of brainstorming activity is also very versatile and can be used at any stage during the workshop to generate ideas and to

Definitions

Listening to others
Giving advice
Not advising
Helping others to help themselves
Problem solving
Handling difficult situations
Sometimes confronting others

Skills

Reflecting back
Asking questions
Only listening
Talking appropriately
Learning to share

Other issues

Difficult!
Not for all nurses
Only for professionals
Everyone should be able to counsel
What everyone does anyway
Hard to define
Not taught in nurse training
Taught to most nurses now

Figure 14.1 An example of sorting in brainstorming

stimulate discussion. It is important, though, that it is not *overused* or it can stimulate groans of 'not brainstorming *again*!' from group participants.

Activity six: an alternative to both of the above methods is that of giving out a prepared handout for discussion. This simply means that the facilitator comes prepared with a single page handout that contains headings, which the group then discusses with the facilitator. At the beginning of the workshop, suitable headings include:

- Definitions of counselling
- Counselling in nursing
- What are counselling skills
- Are you an effective counsellor?
- What do you need from this workshop?

This is probably the safest introduction but hardly the most creative or interactive. It can be useful with groups who are not used to experiential learning activities and who are uncertain about their new role as workshop participants.

Activities which develop listening skills

After an introductory discussion on the nature of counselling and after some formal input from the facilitator, it is usually time to focus on the skills of counselling. The first activities described here are those that focus on the most fundamental and important skill in counselling – listening.

Activity seven: this is a variant on the pairs activity described above. Participants are invited to pair off and to nominate one of each pair as A and the other as B. A then talks to B (about anything) while B does not listen. After five minutes, roles are reversed and B talks to A while A does not listen.

After the second five minute period, the group reconvenes and there is a discussion about what it was like not to be listened to. The exercise is then repeated with each partner listening to the other. Again, the first round of the activity is for five minutes, while A talks to B (who listens). After five minutes, roles are reversed and A listens to B. Again, it should be emphasized that this is not a conversation but an exercise in listening. After the second phase of the activity, the group reconvenes and the facilitator helps the group to identify the key issues in the skill of listening to another person. It is here that it is useful to discuss Egan's (1991) behavioural aspects of counselling (as discussed in more detail in an earlier chapter. They are:

- Sit squarely
- Maintain an open position
- Lean slightly towards the other person
- Maintain comfortable eye contact
- Relax.

As another activity, group participants can be invited to pair off again and to practise listening to each other while observing Egan's listening behaviours.

Activity eight: this activity is one that is carried out with the whole group. It is one that Carl Rogers, the founder of client-centred therapy used to use as a training exercise (Kirschenbaum, 1979). A group discussion on any topic (but preferably one related to counselling) is held. The only ground rule for the discussion is that if anyone wants to contribute to it, they must first summarize what the person before them has said, to that person's satisfaction. Thus, the discussion might sound like this:

> 'Peter said that he thought counselling was difficult in nursing because of the time factor. I think we *could* do counselling if we wanted to. It's a question of sorting out your priorities. I think primary nursing will make a difference. It helps you to think about what you really want to do to help the patient you're looking after . . .'.
>
> 'Sam is saying that she thinks primary nursing can help on the counselling front because it can help you sort out your priorities. I agree with that but only if *everybody* wants to do primary nursing properly. Too many sisters and charge nurses think that primary nursing is just patient allocation. I think its a lot more than that . . .'.
>
> 'Ali said that she thinks that a lot of nurses get confused about what primary nursing is and that they don't like it very much because its threatening ... .'.
>
> 'No . . . that's not quite what I said . . .'.
>
> 'Sorry . . . You said that lots of sisters and charge nurses think that primary nursing is the same as patient allocation . . . I think that primary nurses are in just the right position to work as counsellors . . .'.

The activity takes some getting used to and can be frustrating for some people. It does sharpen up listening skills considerably and is worth using at different times throughout the life of a counselling skills workshop.

Activity nine: finally in this short selection of listening exercises, a different sort of exercise altogether. Group participants are invited to leave the room and to go and sit in a crowded area somewhere in the college or building. They are then asked merely to watch people listening to each other and to note the behaviours that people use as they listen. After a 15 minute period, they return to the main group and discuss what they have seen and heard. The objective is not to ask students to eavesdrop but to ask them to *observe* other people listening. One of the best places to do this is a cafeteria or staff restaurant. Again, Egan's SOLER behaviours can be brought into the discussion that follows.

Activities which encourage client-centred counselling skills

This book has discussed many of the skills of client-centred counselling, although it has also acknowledged the limitations of the approach. As a simple and non-invasive method, though, it is an important one. These are some activities that can be used to develop basic client-centred skills.

Activity ten: again, the pairs format can be used to advantage. In this case, the pairs take it in turns to use either one or a range of the following client-centred skills:

- Open questions
- Empathy building
- Checking for understanding
- Reflection.

After each pair has had a turn in the roles of client and counsellor, the group reconvenes and a discussion is held about the various skills.

Two procedures can be used in this format. Participants can be invited to *role play* counsellor and client. In this case, it is an 'as if' situation: both parties are trying to imagine what it would be like to use the skills in real life. The other option is that both participants stay themselves and one uses the skills while the other talks about real life issues. In this case, the activity is not *role play* but true *skills rehearsal*.

This is an important distinction to make and one to clarify at the outset.

Activity eleven: a variant on the above activity is to encourage a group discussion in which participants use the client-centred skills freely as part of that discussion. Thus, the discussion may sound like this:

> *First participant*: 'You sound as though you are finding the workshop a bit tough. What is it that you find difficult?
> *Second participant*: 'Well, it's the activities that are the most difficult. I've never been good at this sort of thing . . .'
> *Third participant*: 'You don't think you're good at role play and things?'
> *Second participant*: 'Oh, I don't mind them really, but they do make you feel a bit uncomfortable . . .'

It is recommended that the discussion be allowed to run for about 30 minutes after which a full discussion is held about the nature and application of client-centred skills. This activity is also useful if participants are keen to develop *facilitation* skills as well as counselling skills.

Activity twelve: another option is to invite participants to leave the room and to go away and strike up conversations with other people, using the client-centred skills as part of those conversations. After a given period, they agree to return to the larger group and discuss their experiences. These real life exercises and activities can be particularly useful for reinforcing how counselling skills really can be used in everyday life.

Activities to use at the end of learning session

In order to draw the threads of the day together and to end the day on a communal note, it is helpful to engage in an activity in which everyone takes part. Here are three such activities.

Activity thirteen: first, a simple pair of rounds. In the first round, each participant, in turn, says what he or she liked least about the day. Comments can be about any aspect of the day and the comments are not discussed: they are taken to be that person's personal view of what has happened. If a person has nothing to say, he or she says 'pass'. In the second round, each person in turn says what he or she liked most about the day: again about any aspect of the day. Once the last person has spoken in the second round, the day finishes.

Activity fourteen: a variant on the above activity is to invite each person in turn to state three things that they have learned from the day. As in the previous activity, there should be no discussion about what participants say following this round. The idea, here, is that if a discussion ensues, participants may feel that in subsequent rounds, they have to modify what they feel in order that they avoid having what they say discussed by the whole group. The short, relatively silent round is often the best format.

Activity fifteen: another way of ending the day is to have an 'unfinished business' session. This is ten minutes put aside at the end of the day in which people can make statements about anything that has been said or done during the day or about anything that is on their mind at the time. A useful preamble to this activity is for the facilitator to say:

> 'It may be helpful if you share with the group anything that is on your mind – anything that you might otherwise take with you or about which you might say afterwards: "I wish I'd said something about that!" . . .'.

Again, it is probably better that no discussion takes place during or after the unfinished business session. There are exceptions to this rule. In some cases, a participant may *ask* for a particular issue to be discussed in which case it would be rather odd not to take up the request.

Activities for ending a counselling workshop

Finally, the counselling workshop will end. It is helpful if some sort of ritual is carried out to mark the end of the meeting of participants and three such rituals are described here.

Activity sixteen: first, the slow round. This is a round that is taken at a leisurely pace and in which each participant is encouraged to share with the group any thoughts or feelings that he or she has had about the group's time together: negative and positive. Anything is allowed here and the disclosures should be as frank and as full as is possible.

Again, a decision has to be made about whether or not a discussion will take place about the issues that are raised. As a general rule, it is usually better not to have a discussion.

Activity seventeen: another way of ending a workshop is to have a group hug. Some people feel very strongly about such activities and this one is only for those who are happy with a fair degree of physical contact with others. No one should feel compelled to take part and the facilitator should use his or her discretion about whether or not it is appropriate to suggest the group hug.

Group members stand in a close circle and each person puts his arms around the people on the other side. The group then stays in this position for a few minutes, preferably in silence. Alternatively, people in the circle can share their feelings about each other or the workshop.

Activity eighteen: finally, it is possible to hold a more prolonged unfinished business session at the close of a workshop. Here, an hour is put aside for frank and open disclosure of anything that group participants want to raise. Here, it is important that each person decides for him or herself whether or not they want a discussion of the issue that it raised. This can be a powerful way of self and peer assessment and evaluation.

These are some of the issues to consider when planning to run a counselling skills workshop for nurses. They are also things to think about for the person who is considering going on a counselling skills course and who wonders what such a course may be like. This book has offered a model of counselling. It is a simple and usable model which encourages you to think carefully about how you plan and develop your counselling skills. Now it is over to you for in the end, what really counts, is how counselling is *practised*.

Questions for reflection and discussion

- Who have been good facilitators for you?
- Could you run a counselling skills workshop?
- What are the negative aspects of facilitation?

15

Specific problems and some solutions

Counselling, like life itself, rarely runs as smoothly as it does in books. In this final chapter, some typical and specific problems in counselling are highlighted. Some solutions to these problems are also offered. How you *actually* deal with such problems will depend upon many things: the context; the relationships; the time that you have; your personality and so forth. The solutions offered here merely highlight some of the ways that there are of dealing with the issues. Also, the solutions draw attention, once again, to the basic principles described in Chapter 1.

The problems are mostly written as a series of 'What if?' questions and they are followed, directly, by some ways of coping. You are asked to read through the solutions and decide for yourself whether or not any one particular solution is the one that *you* would choose. If you find yourself disagreeing with all of the solutions, try to identify what you would do if you were faced with the particular problem. Once again, it helps if you can discuss these problems and the solutions that I have suggested. As with most things, there are rarely right and wrong answers in this domain. Human beings are infinitely complicated and variable and it is rarely possible to offer *the* answer to a given problem.

Use this chapter, too, to review your thoughts about counselling. Think about how likely or unlikely it would be that you could find yourself facing the problems in this chapter. Think, too, about what other difficulties you can anticipate and think about how you might deal with such problems.

One of the clearest and simplest ways of coping with problems is to self-disclose your feelings or thoughts. For example, when you find yourself stuck and do not know what to say, then consider disclosing to the client that you feel that way. Sometimes, we feel that this is unprofessional. We feel that we should have the answers. However, to share our own thoughts in this way is to acknowledge that we, too, are human. Such disclosure sometimes helps to reveal the next move. It is as though the self-disclosure clears the air and allows the relationship to develop further.

These are the problems and some suggested solutions.

1 What if I have to counsel children? Do the principles suggested in this book apply?

Most of the principles in this book apply to counselling children, especially the sections on the client-centred approach. It is suggested, though, that counselling children calls for additional skills not discussed in this book. As a rule, though, the main point applies: listen, listen and listen some more. Other issues that need to be borne in mind when talking to children in a health care setting, include the following:

- Remember that many small children will only talk to you through their parent. They will probably have been told not to talk to strangers and there is no obvious reason to assume that you are not a stranger.
- Allow the child to decide on where he or she sits in relation to you and let him or her decide on the distance between you.
- Think carefully about the 'language register' that you use. Explain what you mean and avoid jargon.
- Believe what the child tells you. He or she is trying to communicate and needs to be believed if the conversation is going to work.
- Do not patronize or talk down. Do not laugh at any of the comical things that the child may say. It does not help them and does not enhance your own credibility.
- Take your time and let the child do the talking. Do not be too anxious to do counselling with the child. Avoid, particularly, acting as a psychotherapist unless you have particular training in this field.
- Be normal. Talk to the child in a normal way. You do not have to adopt a special voice for talking to children nor do you have to try to mimic their language style or use their catchwords or phrases.
- Talk through play. Often, the child will talk more freely if you are both involved in a game.

2 What if the person I am counselling tells me something that embarrasses me?

Your best bet, here, is to allow yourself to be embarrassed. If you are prone to blushing, it is unlikely that any amount of control will do any good. Also, the acknowledgement and personal acceptance that you are embarrassed tends to show that you are human. You may also find it useful to acknowledge to the client that you are embarrassed. This issue of self-disclosure is sometimes a difficult one, but it is one that can lead to further discussion about why the client has chosen such an embarrassing thing to discuss with you and why *you* are embarrassed and what normally happens when the client discusses this sort of issue.

3 What if I find myself disliking the patient I am counselling?

One thing you can do, here, is to ask yourself, 'whom does this person remind me of?' This is sometimes known as disassociation. When we meet someone for the first time, they sometimes remind us of a person we knew in the past and either liked or disliked. Sometimes, this process is very obvious to us and we think, 'He reminds me of Andrew!' At other times, the association is hidden from us and we just have an odd feeling about the other person. Searching your memory for who this person is linked with in your mind can help to clear the association.

If this does not work, there is always the possibility that you do not like the person! Obviously, we cannot always hope to like the person who comes to us for counselling any more than we can like all our other patients. If this is the case, two possibilities occur: you ask someone else to talk to the client, or you push ahead and carry on with your counselling, acknowledging, to yourself, that you do not like him or her. It is not a necessary prerequisite of counselling that you like your client, although it usually helps.

4 What if the other person tells me they have done something illegal?

This puts you in a difficult position for unlike people in the church or in the Samaritan organization, you do not and cannot offer total confidentiality. The best way of dealing with this is to avoid the likelihood of its happening by *avoiding* offering total confidentiality in the first place. If the client is aware that what is being talked about is not necessarily for your ears only and that some things may have to be discussed with colleagues, then if such a disclosure is made, it becomes clear to both of you that the information must be passed on. With such an occurrence, it would be appropriate to talk to a senior nurse about what has been disclosed to you.

If you *have* offered total confidentiality, the situation is more complicated. The fact that you *know* about what has happened makes you a potential *accomplice* to the fact. You then have the choice of either keeping the information to yourself and maintaining confidentiality or breaking the confidentiality contract and talking to a senior nurse about it. While this must always be a question of personal ethical choice, if the illegal act was likely to put the client or other people at risk, then on the principle of utilitarianism (or what is right is that which creates the greatest happiness for the greatest number), I would be inclined to tell another person. By telling you about an illegal act, the client has displaced some of the responsibility for the act onto you.

5 What if I find myself attracted to the person I am counselling?

Again, a number of options open up. First, you could acknowledge to yourself that this is happening. This is an important step for it is easy to avoid such self-awareness. Second, you could accept the fact and work on through it, trying, where possible, to ignore the fact. Finding someone attractive is not an unusual state of affairs nor is it one that must, necessarily, be acted upon. Finally, you could consider disclosing the fact to the client, though before you do this, you should consider your motives for so doing. There can be no situation in which *acting* upon your feelings could be apptopriate, given that you are a professional person offering a professional relationship.

6 What if the client's problems turn out to be my problems?

This will often be the case! Carl Rogers (1967) makes the point that, 'what is most personal is most general'. The things that *you* worry about and keep to yourself are probably the same sorts of things that *I* worry about and tend to hide. When you find yourself identifying with the client's problems, acknowledge the fact to yourself and press on. Again, you may have to decide whether or not to disclose the issue to the client but, you should consider what your motives might be in doing this. If the problem under discussion is an *insurmountable* or painful one for you, you may have to make the decision to refer the client to another person for help.

7 What if I get bored?

This is an odd, but fairly common phenomenon. It is not unusual to find yourself yawning during some sessions with a client! At least three things may be happening here; you are bored; you are very tired or the client's voice is soporific; or the client is talking about something that is important to you but about which you do not want to listen. If the first two apply, then asking questions or generally becoming more active in the conversation can help. If the last one applies, you may need to talk your own problems through with a colleague. You may also need to wake up a little and to listen really to what the client is saying.

8 What if I find counselling too much to cope with?

Two options open up here. If you are able to and it does not stress the client too much, you can discuss the fact with the client and work towards his or her seeing another person. If you cannot discuss it directly, then go and see a senior colleague or a more experienced counsellor and seek advice about referring on.

9 What if I get burnt out?

Burnout, the negative effects of long exposure to other people's problems, is a potential problem for anyone working in the caring professions. It is also a particular threat to counsellors who often work on their own and hold all sorts of problems in confidence. Here are some things you can do both to avoid and deal with burnout:

- Set up a supervision relationship with another counsellor. Have somebody with whom you can discuss what happens between you and the client. Tell the client, at the start of the relationship that you are going to have this supervision and that it will benefit you both.
- Do not take on too many clients. This is an obvious one but it is sometimes quite difficult to say 'no' to people who are obviously distressed. Do stay within the limits of your time and emotional energy.
- Take regular breaks. Make sure that you use all of your holidays and then have a complete break from the nursing world. Do not use holiday to go to conferences and workshops if you are also doing a lot of counselling.
- Learn practical ways of coping with stress. There are various books on this topic which can help you learn to plan your time more effectively and to cope with job related stress (Bond, 1986; Burnard, 1991c).

10 What if the client starts arriving late or missing appointments?

Always discuss this with the client when it happens over a period of time. It may be a signal that the client wants to stop counselling and does not know how to tell you. It may also be a sign that he or she is finding the whole process painful. Talking about lateness or non-attendance can be a gentle way into such issues.

11 Are the principles of AIDS counselling the same as those described in this model?

The general principles described here apply to all types of counselling. However, AIDS counselling will call upon a range of client-centred and information and advice-giving skills. It will also demand that nurses have clear and up-to-date information about AIDS and HIV. Also, AIDS counselling is not one homogeneous sort of counselling. A number of different sorts of client groups can be identified under the heading, including, at least, the following:

- People who are anxious about AIDS and want to avoid it
- Those who think they may have AIDS and want to know what to do next
- Those who are thinking about being tested and do not know whether or not they should
- Those who have been tested and are found to be HIV positive
- Those who are tested and found not to be HIV positive
- Those who have been HIV positive for some time and who are worried about full blown AIDS
- Those who have full blown AIDS.

There is now a large literature on AIDS counselling and the nurse who is anticipating working in this field is advised to read some of this and to consider seriously specific training in the field. Important titles in this field include the following (although it should be borne in mind that titles are constantly being updated and revised):

- Bor, R. (1991) The ABC of AIDS counselling. *Nursing Times*, 87 1, 32–35.
- Connor, S. and Kingman, S. (1989) *The search for the virus: the scientific discovery of AIDS and the quest for a cure.* Penguin, Harmondsworth.
- Dilley, J. W., Pies, C. and Helquist, M. (1989) *Face to face: A guide to AIDS counselling.* AIDS Health Project, University of California, San Francisco.
- Miller, C. (1990) *The AIDS Handbook.* Penguin, Harmondsworth.
- Miller, D. (1987) *Living with AIDS and HIV.* Macmillan, London.
- Pratt, R. J. (1988) *AIDS: a strategy for nursing care.* Arnold, London.
- Pye, M., Kapila, M., Buckley, G. and Cunningham, D. (eds). (1989) *Local AIDS Programmes in the UK.* Longman, London.
- Sketchley, J. (1989) Counselling people affected by HIV and AIDS. In *Handbook of counselling in Britain* W. Dryden, D. Charles-Edwards and R. Woolfe eds). Tavistock/Routledge, London.
- Welch, J. (1990) *Looking after people with late HIV disease.* The Pattern Press in association with the Lisa Sainsbury Foundation, London.

Also, there is a variety of teaching packages and videos that are available for hire to enable people to learn more about AIDS and HIV. Examples of materials available at the time of writing include the following, although it should be appreciated that the field is changing rapidly and teaching and learning materials are being updated all the time:

- *AIDS teaching pack* 1990 TACADE – Teachers Advisory Council on Drug & Alcohol Education, 3rd Floor, Furness House, Trafford Road, Salford, M5 2XJ
- *Teaching about AIDS and HIV* 1988 Health Education Authority, Hamilton House, Mabledon Place, London
- *Underground AIDS* 1989 Metro Pictures Limited, 79 Wardour Street, London
- *AIDS/HIV - a woman's issue* 1989 Metro Pictures Limited, 79 Wardour Street, London
- *Escape AIDS* Jordanhill College Publications, Jordanhill College of Education, 76 Southbrae Drive, Glasgow, G13 1PP
- *AIDS for training* 1989 Albany Video Distribution, Battersea Studios, Television Centre, Thackeray Road, London, SW8 3TW
- *AIDS and you: an illustrated guide* 1988 BMA Library, Film & Video Services, BMA House, Tavistock Place, London, WC1H 9JP

Sketchley (1989), in a useful and informative paper about counselling people affected by HIV and AIDS, suggests that there are three elements to AIDS counselling:

- Education
- Advice
- Psychosocial counselling.

Sketchley suggests that these three elements overlap in the AIDS counselling process. In this respect, AIDS counselling is an example of the eclectic approach advocated in this book: a combination of helping the client to make decisions for him or herself, the ability to give clear and appropriate advice when this is required and the skill of undertaking the appropriate education and training roles necessary in all aspects of nursing. It must be repeated, though, that in AIDS counselling, it is essential that up-to-date information about safe sex, prevention and living with AIDS is known to all those who work alongside people with AIDS. In *this* respect, AIDS counselling is a special case in counselling.

In a recent study I found that health professionals felt that all nurses should have a thorough knowledge and understanding of AIDS and related disorders, although they did not feel that all nurses need to train as AIDS counsellors (Burnard, 1991a). It would seem imperative that nurses *do* know enough about AIDS to be able to offer either appropriate advice or to be able to refer on appropriately.

Appendix 1: useful addresses

There are numerous colleges and organizations that offer training in counselling. Listed below are some that will be useful as a starting point to thinking about becoming a counsellor or developing your skills or as places to refer patients and clients to.

Alcoholics Anonymous
PO Box 1
Stonebow House
Stonebow
York
YO1 2NJ

Asian Family Counselling Service
Equity Chambers
40 Picadilly
Bradford
BD1 3NN

Association of Humanistic Psychology Practitioners
14 Mornington Grove
London
E3 4NS

British Association for Dramatherapists
The Old Mill
Tolpuddle
Dorchester
Dorset
DT2 7EX

British Pregnancy Advisory Service
Austy Manor
Wootton Wawen
Solihull
B95 6BX

British Association for Counselling
37a Sheep Street
Rugby
Warwickshire
CV21 3BX

British Association for Psychotherapists
121 Hendon Lane
London

Brook Advisory Centres
153a East street
London
SE17 2SD

Cancer Help Centre
Grove Road
Cornwallis Grove
Clifton
Bristol
BS8 4PG

Catholic Marriage Advisory Council
1 Blythe Mews
Blythe Road
London
W14 0NW

Centre for Counselling and Psychotherapy Education
21 Lancaster Road
London
W11 1QL

Centre for Personal Construct Psychology
132 Warwick Way
London
SW1 4JD

CHAT
Royal College of Nursing
20 Cavendish square
London
W1H 0AB

Childline
Freepost 1111
London
N1 0BR

CRUSE
126 Sheen Road
Richmond
TW9 1UR

Family Planning Association
27–35 Mortimer Street
London
W1N 7RJ

Gale Centre for Creative Therapy
Whitakers Way
Loughton
Essex
IG10 1SQ

Gay Bereavement Project
Unitarian Rooms
Hoop Lane
London
NW11 8BS

Human Potential Resource Group
Department of Educational Studies
University of Surrey
Guildford
Surrey
GU2 5HX

Incest Crisis Line
PO Box 32
Northolt
Middlesex
UB5 4JC

National Children's Homes Carelines
85 Highbury Park
London
N5 1UD

Institute of Psychotherapy and Social Studies
5 Lake House
South Hill Park
London
NW3 2SH

Institute of Group Analysis
1 Daleham Gardens
London
NW3 5BY

Institute of Family Therapy
43 New Cavendish Street
London

Jewish Marriage Guidance Council
23 Ravenshurst Avenue
London
NW4 4EE

London Institute for the Study of Human Sexuality
10 Warwick Road
Earl's Court
London
SW5 9UH

MIND
22 Harley Street
London
W1 2ED

Minster Centre
57 Minster Road
London
NW2 3SH

National AIDS Helpline
PO Box 1577
Camden Town
London
NW1 3DW

National Step-Family Association
72 Willesden Lane
London
NW6 7TA

NSPCC
67 Saffron Hill
London
EC1N 8RS

Pregnancy Advisory Service
11–13 Charlotte Street
London
W1P 1HD

RELATE
Herbert Gray College
Little Church Street
Rugby
Warwickshire
CV21 3AP

Richmond Fellowship for Community Mental Health
8 Addison Road
London
W14 8DL

Tavistock Institute of Marital Studies
Tavistock Centre
120 Belsize Lane
London
NW3 5BA

Terrence Higgins Trust
BM AIDS
London
WC1N 3XX

The Samaritans
17 Uxbridge Road
Slough
SL1 1SN

Westminster Pastoral Foundation
23 Kensington Square
London
W8 5HN

Women's Health and Reproductive Rights Information Centre
52–54 Featherstone Street
London
EC1Y 8RT

Appendix 2: counselling skills assessment rating scale

You can use the rating scale shown in Figure A2.1 to assess your own counselling skills in various ways:

- Use it periodically to monitor your skills development
- Use it in a group setting to compare and contrast various skills in the group
- Use it at the beginning, middle and end of a counselling skills workshop to check progress.

Counselling skill	1st rating (1–10)	2nd rating (1–10)	3rd rating (1–10)
	Date:	Date:	Date:
1 Introducing self			
2 Discussing a contract			
3 Exploring issues			
4 Identifying priorities			
5 Helping with feelings			
6 Exploring alternatives			
7 Ending the relationship			
9 Questioning			
10 Reflecting			
11 Demonstrating empathy			
12 Checking for understanding			
13 Demonstrating personal warmth			
14 Demonstrating unconditional positive regard			
15 Demonstrating genuineness			
16 Demonstrating knowledge of counselling theory			
17 Demonstrating self-awareness			

KEY: 1 = Very unskilled . . . . . 10 = Very skilled

Figure A2.1 Counselling skills assessment scale

References

Alberti, R. E. and Emmons, M. L. (1982) *Your perfect right: a guide to assertive living*. Impact, San Luis Obispo, California.

Allport, G. (1984) *Live and Learn*. Harper & Row, London.

Arnold, E. and Boggs, K. (1989) *Interpersonal relationships: professional communication skills for nurses*. Saunders, Philadelphia.

Bond, M. (1986) *Stress and self-awareness: a guide for nurses*. Heinemann, London.

Bowlby, J. (1975) *Separation*. Penguin, Harmondsworth.

Buber, M. (1958) *I and Thou*. Scribner, New York.

Burnard, P. (1989) *Teaching interpersonal skills: an experiential handbook for health professionals*. Chapman & Hall, London.

Burnard, P. (1990) *Learning human skills: an experiential guide for nurses* 2nd edn. Heinemann, Oxford.

Burnard, P. (1991a) Perceptions of AIDS. *Journal of District Nursing*, 9 12, 24–26.

Burnard, P. (1991b) *Experiential learning in action*. Avebury, Aldershot.

Burnard, P. (1991c) *Coping with stress in the health professions*. Chapman & Hall, London.

Burnard, P. and Chapman, C. R. (1988) *Professional and ethical issues in nursing: the code of professional conduct*. Wiley, Chichester.

Burnard, P. and Morrison, P. (1988) Nurses' perceptions of their interpersonal skills: a descriptive study using six category intervention analysis. *Nurse Education Today*, 8, 266–272.

Burnard, P. and Morrison, P. (1989) Counselling attitudes in community pyschiatric nurses. *Community Psychiatric Nursing Journal*, 9 5, 26–29

Campbell, A. (1984) *Moderated love*. SPCK, London.

Claxton, G. (1984) *Live and learn: an introduction to the psychology of growth and change in everyday life*. Harper and Row, London.

Cox, M. (1978) *Structuring the therapeutic process*. Pergamon, London.

Egan, G. (1990) *The skilled helper: a systematic approach to effective helping*, 4th edn. Brooks/Cole, Pacific Grove, California.

Eliot, T. S. (1965) *Selected poems*. Faber, London

Frankl, V. E. (1975) Paradoxical intention and dereflection: a logotherapeutic technique. *Psychotherapy: Theory, Research and Practice*. **12**, 3, 226–237.

Gendlin, E. (1981) *Focussing*. Bantam, New York.

Hales-Tooke, J. (1989) Focussing in therapy: focussing in life: self and society. *European Journal of Humanistic Psychology*, **XVII**, 6, 113–116.
Hawkins, P. and Shohet, R. (1989) *Supervision in the helping professions*. Open University Press, Milton Keynes.
Heron, J. (1989) *Six category intervention analysis*, 2nd edn. Human Potential Resource Group, University of Surrey, Guildford, Surrey.
Heron, J. (1990) *Helping the client*. Sage, London.
Jourard, S. (1967) *The transparent self*. Van Nostrand, New York.
Kalisch, B. J. (1971) Strategies for developing nurses' empathy. *Nursing Outlook*, **19**, 11, 714–717.
Kelly, G. (1955) *The psychology of personal constructs*; Vol 1 and 2. Norton, New York.
Kelly, G. (1969) *The autobiography of a theory. Clinical psychology and personality:* Selected Papers of George Kelly, B. A. Maher (ed). Wiley, New York.
Kirschenbaum, H. (1979) *On becoming Carl Rogers*. Dell, New York.
Lowen, A. (1967) *The betrayal of the body*. Macmillan, New York.
Lowen, A. and Lowen, L. (1977) *The way to vibrant health: a manual of bioenergetic exercises*. Harper and Row, New York.
Luft, J. (1967) *Of human interaction: the Johari model*. Mayfield, Palo Alto, California.
Mayeroff, M. (1972) *On caring*. Harper and Row, New York.
Morrison, P. and Burnard, P. (1989) Students' and trained nurses' perceptions of their own interpersonal skills: a report and comparison. *Journal of Advanced Nursing*, **14**, 321–329.
Morrison, P. and Burnard, P. (1991) *Caring and communicating: the interpersonal relationship in nursing*. Macmillan, London.
Murgatroyd, S. (1985) *Counselling and helping*. Methuen, London.
Ornstein, R. E. (1975) *The psychology of consciousness*. Penguin, Harmondsworth.
Patterson, C. H. (1985) *The therapeutic relationship: foundations for an eclectic psychotherapy*. Brooks/Cole, Pacific Grove, California.
Perls, F. (1969) *Gestalt therapy verbatim*. Real People Press, Lafayette, California.
Quilliam, S. and Grove-Stephensen, I. (1991) *The best counselling guide*. Thorsons, London.
Reich, W. (1949) *Character analysis*. Simon and Schuster, New York.
Rogers, C. R. (1951) *Client-centred therapy*. Constable, London.
Rogers, C. R. (1967) *On becoming a person*. Constable, London.
Rogers, C. R. (1983) *Freedom to learn for the eighties*. Merill, Columbus, Ohio.
Sartre, J-P. (1954) *Being and nothingness*. Philosophical Library, New York.
Schulman, D. (1982) *Intervention in human services: A guide to skills and knowledge*, 3rd edn. C. V. Mosby, St Louis, Missouri.
Sketchley, J. (1989) Counselling people affected by HIV and AIDS. In *Handbook of counselling in Britain*. (W. Dryden, D. Charles-Edwards and R. Woolfe eds). Tavistock/Routledge, London

Sullivan, H. S. (1955) *The psychiatric interview*. Harper and Row, New York.
Synder, M. (1985) *Independent nursing functions*. Wiley, New York.
Vonnegut, K. (1968) *Mother night*. Gollancz, London.
Wilkinson, J. and Canter, S. (1982) *Social skills training manual: assessment programme design and management of training*. Wiley, Chichester.

Bibliography

As an aid to using this bibliography, I have indicated publications that I feel to be essential reading with an asterisk.

Alberti, R. E. and Emmons, M.L. (1982) *Your perfect right: a guide to assertive living*, 4th edn. Impact Publishers, San Luis, California.

Allan, J. (1989) *How to develop your personal management skills*. Kogan Page, London.

Baruth, L. G. (1987) *An introduction to the counselling profession*. Prentice Hall, Englewood Cliffs, New Jersey.

Belkin, G. S. (1984) *Introduction to counselling*. Brown, Dubuque, Iowa.

Bower, S. A. and Bower, G. H. (1976) *Asserting yourself*. Addison Wesley, Reading, Mass.

Broome, A. (1990) *Managing change*. Macmillan, London.

Brown, D. and Srebalus, D. J. (1988) *An introduction to the counselling process*. Prentice Hall, Philadelphia, PA

*Buber, M. (1958) *I and thou*. Scribner, New York.

Bugental, E. K. and Bugental, J. F. T. (1984) Dispiritedness: a new perspective on a familiar state. *Journal of Humanistic Psychology*, **24**, 1, 49–67.

*Burnard, P. (1989) *Counselling skills for health professionals*. Chapman & Hall, London.

Burnard, P. (1990) *Learning human skills: an experiential guide for nurses*, 2nd edn. Heinemann, London.

Burnard, P. (1991) *Coping with stress in the health professions: a practical guide*. Chapman & Hall, London.

Burnard, P. (1991) *Effective communication skills for health professionals*. Chapman & Hall, London.

*Campbell, A. (1984) *Moderated love*. SPCK, London.

Campbell, A. (1984) *Paid to care?* SPCK, London.

*Claxton, G. (1984) *Live and learn: an introduction to the psychology of growth and change in everyday life*. Harper and Row, London.

Cox, M. (1978) *Structuring the therapeutic process*. Pergamon, London.

Dickson, A. (1985) *A woman in your own right: assertiveness and you*. Quartet Books, London.

Dixon, D. N. and Glover, J. A. (1984) *Counselling: a problem solving approach*. Wiley, Chichester.

*Dryden, W., Charles-Edwards, D. and Woolfe, R. (1989) *Handbook of counselling in Britain*. Tavistock/Routledge, London.

*Egan, G. (1990) *The skilled helper: a systematic approach to effective helping*, 4th edn. Brooks/Cole, Pacific Grove, California.

*Frankl, V. E. (1969) *The will to meaning*. World Publishing Co, New York.

Frankl, V. E. (1978) *The unheard cry for meaning*. Simon and Schuster, New York.

Gibson, R. L. and Mitchell, M. H. (1986) *Introduction to counselling and guidance*. Collier Macmillan, London

*Halmos, P. (1965) *The faith of the counsellors*. Constable, London.

Hawkins, P. and Shohet, R. (1989) *Supervision and the helping professions*. Open University Press, Milton Keynes.

Herinck, R. (ed) (1980) *The psychotherapy handbook*. New American Library, New York.

*Heron, J. (1990) *Helping the client*. Sage, London.

Howard, G. S., Nance, D. W. and Meyers, P. (1987) *Adaptive counselling and therapy: a systematic approach to selecting effective treatments*. Jossey Bass, San Francisco, California.

Ivey, A. E. (1987) *Counselling and psychotherapy: skills, theories and practice*. Prentice Hall International, London.

Johnson, D.W. (1972) *Reaching out*. Prentice Hall, Englewood Cliffs, New Jersey.

*Jourard, S. (1964) *The transparent self*. Van Nostrand, Princeton, New Jersey.

*Kopp, S. (1974) *If you meet the Buddha on the road, kill him: a modern pilgrimage through myth, legend and psychotherapy*. Sheldon Press, London.

Kottler, J. A. and Brown, R. W. (1985) *Introduction to therapeutic counselling*. Brooks-Cole, Monterey, California

Leech, K. (1986) *Spirituality and pastoral care*. Sheldon Press, London.

Marshall, E. K. and Kurtz, P. D. (eds) (1982) *Interpersonal helping skills: a guide to training methods, programs and resources*. Jossey Bass, San Francisco, California.

Marson, S. (ed) (1990) *Managing people*. Macmillan, London.

*Morrison, P. and Burnard, P. (1990) *Caring and communicating: the interpersonal relationship in nursing*. Macmillan, London.

Morsund, J. (1985) *The process of counselling and therapy*. Prentice Hall, Englewood Cliffs, New Jersey.

Munro, A., Manthei, B. and Small, J. (1988) *Counselling: the skills of problem-solving*. Routledge, London.

*Murgatroyd, S. (1986) *Counselling and helping*. British Psychological Society and Methuen, London.

Murgatroyd, S. and Woolfe, R. (1982) *Coping with crisis-understanding and helping persons in need*. Harper and Row, London.

Myerscough, P. R. (1989) *Talking with patients: a basic clinical skill*. Oxford Medical Publications, Oxford.

*Nelson-Jones, R. (1981) *The theory and practice of counselling psychology*. Holt Rhinehart and Winston, London.

Nelson-Jones, R. (1984) *Personal responsibility: counselling and therapy: an integrative approach*. Harper and Row, London.
Nelson-Jones, R. (1988) *Practical counselling and helping skills: helping clients to help themselves*. Cassell, London.
Nichols, K. and Jenkinson, J. (1990) *Leading a support group*. Chapman & Hall, London.
Porritt, L. (1990) *Interaction strategies: an introduction for health professionals*, 2nd edn. Churchill Livingstone, Edinburgh.
Priestly, P., McQuire, J., Flegg, D., Hemsley, V. and Welham, D. (1978) *Social skills and personal problem solving*. Tavistock, London.
Quilliam, S. and Grove-Stephensen, I. (1991) *The best counselling guide*. Thorsons, London.
Reddy, M. (1987) *The manager's guide to counselling at work*. Methuen, London.
Rogers, C. R. (1951) *Client-centred therapy*. Constable, London.
*Rogers, C. R. (1967) *On becoming a person*. Constable, London.
Scammell, B. (1990) *Communication skills*. Macmillan, London.
*Shafer, P. (1978) *Humanistic psychology*. Prentice Hall, Englewood Cliffs, New Jersey.
Totton, N. and Edmonston, E. (1988) *Reichian growth work: melting the blocks to life and love*. Prism Press, Bridport.
Tough, A. M. (1982) *International changes: a fresh approach to helping people change*. Cambridge Books, New York.
*Tschudin, V. (1990) *Counselling skills for nurses*. Balliere Tindall, London.
Tshudin, V. and Schober, J. (1990) *Managing yourself*. Macmillan, London.
Wallace, W.A. (1986) *Theories of counselling and psychotherapy: a basic issues approach*. Allyn and Bacon, Boston.
Watkins, J. (1978) *The therapeutic self*. Human Science Press, New York.

Index